COVID-19: A Critical Care Textbook

COVID-19: A Critical Care Textbook

Chris Carter
Senior Lecturer
Birmingham City University
Westbourne Road
Edgbaston
Birmingham
UK

Joy Notter
Professor of Community
Healthcare Studies
Birmingham City University
Westbourne Road
Edgbaston
Birmingham
UK

ELSEVIER

LONDON • NEW YORK • OXFORD • PHILADELPHIA
ST LOUIS • SYDNEY 2022

Notices

Practitioners and researchers must always rely on their own experience and knowledge in evaluating and using any information, methods, compounds or experiments described herein. Because of rapid advances in the medical sciences, in particular, independent verification of diagnoses and drug dosages should be made. To the fullest extent of the law, no responsibility is assumed by Elsevier, authors, editors or contributors for any injury and/or damage to persons or property as a matter of products liability, negligence or otherwise, or from any use or operation of any methods, products, instructions, or ideas contained in the material herein.

ISBN: 978-0-70-208383-9

Content Strategist: Robert Edwards
Content Development Specialist: Andrae Akeh
Publishing Services Manager: Shereen Jameel
Project Manager: Umarani Natarajan
Design: Bridget Hoette
Marketing Manager: Samantha Page

Printed in the United Kingdom

Last digit is the print number: 9 8 7 6 5 4 3 2 1

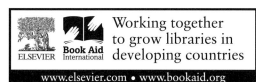

Contents

Foreword

The international community has suffered the largest global public health crisis in over 100 years with the recent COVID-19 pandemic, which has caused significant loss of life. This viral disease has placed considerable strain upon both public health and hospital-based services from the onset. The early phases of the pandemic escalated well beyond expectations, and it is still considered a major problem, with continuing mutations and variance. These are likely to place further waves of pressure on global health systems, causing unimaginable levels of mortality and harm. The international health impact and emerging challenges associated with the long-term consequences of COVID-19, including the emergence of multiorgan problems associated with long COVID-19, will continue to put pressure on health systems and their healthcare workers. In consequence, we will continue to see the effects in physical health, mental health and economic shocks for decades to come.

The response to the pandemic has been varied across the globe, led by national public health agencies in collaboration with the World Health Organization. However, the data reveals that nations have approached the pandemic in different ways, resulting in each country experiencing varied levels of impact in both health and economic terms. What is also evident from all nations is that healthcare workers, including nurses, doctors, scientists and allied health professionals, have worked collaboratively, under extreme pressure, to save lives and improve outcomes. It is important to recognize that globally, many healthcare workers have lost their lives due to COVID-19 infections contracted in the line of duty.

Nations have recognized that the focus, dedication and professionalism of their healthcare workforces will undoubtedly have saved many lives across the globe, and it is hoped that a renewed focus on nations' healthcare systems will be a positive legacy from the COVID-19 pandemic. It is important to recognize that all healthcare workers have contributed to the management of the pandemic, but nursing, as one of the largest workforces in all health systems across the globe, has taken a significant lead in delivering care, undertaking research, providing education and providing leadership at local national and international levels.

In international health systems in the early phases of the pandemic, it was recognized that this novel virus would need significant scientific endeavour to understand its impact on populations and management approaches within community and hospital-based settings. Based upon previous pandemics, it was recognized that there would be a significant burden placed upon hospital services, notably in relation to the requirement for intensive nursing care and complex interventions including invasive/non-invasive ventilation of the most critically injured. Critical care nursing is one of the most technically demanding areas of nursing and care, with years of education and training needed to ensure that the highest quality of care is delivered. During the pandemic, it was evident that in most nations, the number of COVID-19 cases necessitated additional critical care bed capacity. In response to this, in many instances, to prevent services being overwhelmed, additional healthcare workers were trained to work under supervision and deployed into acute services. As the pandemic has evolved, a pattern of waves of infection has emerged, and in consequence, there will be a need for education and training materials in the field for the foreseeable future.

Launched in the Year of Health and Care Workers, designated by WHO as a time to recognize the dedication, sacrifice and contribution of frontline healthcare workers, the authors of this book recognize the need for different levels of information and have worked with frontline nurses to rapidly share assimilated experience and evidence in critical care management of COVID-19. Together they have compiled a comprehensive resource for use in the current pandemic and future pandemic management.

This excellent resource will be critical reading for any healthcare worker involved in pandemic management of critical care patients. I am delighted that this collaboration has drawn upon such wide-ranging professional expertise to ensure that current and future generations of healthcare workers are prepared and supported in pandemic management of this magnitude. While it is inevitable that future pandemics will occur, it is essential that we share the lessons learnt to build resilience, knowledge and expertise that will ultimately save lives.

Prof Mark Radford
Chief Nurse
Health Education England

List of contributors

Helen Aedy Critical Care Outreach Nurse, University Hospital Lewisham, Lewisham & Greenwich NHS Trust, London, United Kingdom

Gifty M. Agagah, BSc (Hons). MA Compliance and Regulation Lead, Compliance & Regulation Department, University Hospital Lewisham, Lewisham and Greenwich NHS Trust, London, United Kingdom

Janice Ferreira Senior Staff Nurse, Critical Care Unit, University Hospital Lewisham, Lewisham & Greenwich NHS Trust, London, United Kingdom

June Frankland, DipHE Adult Nursing Deputy Sister, Critical Care Unit, University Hospital Lewisham, Lewisham & Greenwich NHS Trust, London, United Kingdom

Babita Gurung Staff Nurse, University Hospital Lewisham, Lewisham & Greenwich NIIS Trust, London, Unitcd Kingdom

Nguyen Thi Lan Anh Chief of Nursing Department, Bach Mai Hospital, Executive Vice Dean of Nursing & Midwifery Faculty, Hanoi Medical University, Hanoi, Viet Nam

Grace Lao Senior Staff Nurse, University Hospital Lewisham, Lewisham and Greenwich NHS Trust, London, United Kingdom

Michelle Osborn, Dip HE (Adult) BSc (Hons) Deputy Sister, Critical Care Unit, University Hospital Lewisham, Lewisham & Greenwich NHS Trust, London, United Kingdom

Daniel Paschoud Resuscitation Officer, Lewisham & Greenwich NHS Trust, London, United Kingdom

Rosaleeta Reece-Anthony, BSC (Hons) RN(Adult) Critical Care Research Nurse, Critical Care Unit, University Hospital Lewisham, Lewisham & Greenwich NHS Trust, London, United Kingdom

Martine Rooney Matron, Critical Care Unit, University Hospital Lewisham, Lewisham & Greenwich NHS Trust, London, United Kingdom

Alice Sadra, Dip HE (Adult) BSc (Hons) ENB 100 ENB 998 Sister, Critical Care Unit, University Hospital Lewisham, Lewisham & Greenwich NHS Trust, London, United Kingdom

Introduction

The story of epidemics is the story of inequalities. For many countries, during an outbreak, healthcare priorities have to be diverted from other health priorities to focus on the outbreak response. While this is essential, the long-term effects on the healthcare system and local communities need to be recognized. For many nurses there will be a decade of challenges from the COVID-19 pandemic, as it has had an exponential global impact on an already rising demand for health care, an ageing population, a global lack of nurses and climate change. The impact of the combination of all these factors on economic, social and healthcare provision varies across countries, but while each individual healthcare system will adopt its own approach, there are commonalities in nursing practice that transcend borders. Although vaccination programmes are now in progress, it has to be accepted that mutations and variations in COVID-19 may well impact on healthcare provision for the foreseeable future. While it is accepted that there is no one solution, it has also been recognized that nursing practice will have to continually evolve to meet ever-changing needs. It is therefore essential that nurses work together, sharing good practice through the development and maintenance of actual and virtual international communities of practice. One way to do this is to disseminate lessons learnt and ways in which nurses have had to 'think outside the box' of current practice. To support this approach, we have put together a series of chapters based on experiences of frontline nurses during the COVID-19 pandemic.

We are now in a 'new norm', and while in the short term the focus had to be on an immediate response to the pandemic patients, there was inevitably an impact on access to all other services. To give just one example, in the UK alone, it is estimated that transfer of services to cope with the COVID-19 pandemic reduced access to treatment for many cancer patients, which is likely to lead to around 6270 additional deaths [1]. Evidence is gradually emerging that other countries share the same burden of delayed diagnosis and treatment across a range of both communicable and non-communicable diseases [2]. As a result, countries need to work together to develop innovative and sustainable approaches to redress shortages and support the continuance of services. The nature of COVID-19 is such that the unprecedented and sustained rise in patients needing intensive care may recur, with the result that these other crucial services will be further adversely impacted as providers struggle again to maintain usual service need. The epidemiological and public health modelling of the COVID-19 virus suggests that it will follow a wave format, and that over the next few years healthcare systems must prepare for second, third and potentially fourth waves to accompany the usual cyclic illnesses such as seasonal flu [3].

For nursing, the recent pandemic has highlighted the limited clinical nursing research, although there is a wealth of medical research and publications. This balance must be redressed by nurses and for nurses if nursing as a profession is to be recognized for successful innovation and adaptation in times of challenge, a position that history reveals it has always had.

In terms of critical care, the origins are linked to the polio outbreak in 1952, and COVID-19 has been described as our generation's polio [4], and as with polio, the essential role of critical care nurses has been recognized. Recent events have shown that no one country can fight an outbreak or pandemic on its own. In the past 20 years there have been three outbreaks of respiratory infectious diseases, including severe acute respiratory distress syndrome, Middle East respiratory syndrome (MERS) and more recently, COVID-19. In consequence, sharing of knowledge is essential to understand highly contagious diseases with an unknown or incomplete disease trajectory. While the main emphasis of this book is on severe Covid-19 disease, evidence has shown that there is an increasing incidence of coronaviruses in the livestock animal population, which may pose challenges in the future if these are also, able to transfer to humans [5]. Therefore, we believe that the themes in this text will be relevant and transferrable to other infectious disease outbreaks such as cholera, Ebola, and other coronaviruses.

Although critical care tends to be delivered within intensive care units, traditionally acute and critically ill patients are found in emergency, acute and community settings throughout the healthcare system. Therefore, staff in all clinical areas need to be able to recognize and respond to clinical deterioration and escalate care in order to facilitate an early admission to critical care or avert inappropriate admissions. The current COVID-19 pandemic has shown that to meet the unprecedented numbers of patients requiring critical care, it was necessary for services to expand capacity to the point where additional nursing staff had to be redeployed into critical care units. Therefore, this book contains valuable information for staff working in emergency departments as well as those based in critical care areas. It will help support those who are redeployed to different areas as they adapt to their new clinical environment and adjusted role.

We believe this is the first book of its type. Written for nurses by nurses, international contributors and nurses from the NHS and higher education who have been involved in the recent COVID-19 pandemic have contributed to sections within this book. We hope this book is useful to both medical planners and nurses involved in major incident preparedness and nursing care.

Chris Carter, Joy Notter

References

[1] Lai A, Pasea L, Banerjee, et al. Estimating excess mortality in people with cancer and multi-morbidity in the COVID-19 emergency. 2020. https://doi.org/10.13140/RG.2.2.34254.82242.

[2] Modesti PA, Wang J, Damasceno A, et al. Indirect implications of COVID-19 prevention strategies on non-communicable diseases. BMC Med 2020;18:256. https://doi.org/10.1186/s12916-020-01723-6.

[3] Rubin R. What happens when COVID-19 collides with flu season? JAMA 2020. https://doi.org/10.1001/jama.2020.15260.

[4] Gibbons K, Ball T. Coronavirus is our generation's polio, says doctor who saved Boris Johnson. 2020. https://www.thetimes.co.uk/edition/news/coronavirus-is-our-generations-polio-says-doctor-who-saved-boris-johnson-w2tk8pth0.

[5] Li H, Liu SM, Yu XH, Tang SL, Tang CK. Coronavirus disease 2019 (COVID-19): current status and future perspectives. Int J Antimicrob Agents 2020;55:105951.

Chapter 1

Pathophysiology of SARS-CoV-2

Chris Carter, Joy Notter

Chapter Outline

In late 2019, the World Health Organization (WHO) was alerted to a series of cases of severe pneumonia of unknown aetiology in Wuhan City in Hubei Province in China. Following investigation, this was identified as a new novel coronavirus. The pathogen was initially named "2019nCoV" by the WHO, and later renamed Severe Acute Respiratory Syndrome Coronavirus 2 (SARS-CoV-2) by the Coronavirus Study Group [1]. The disease was ultimately named coronavirus disease-2019 (COVID-19) [2], and as with other viruses it needs to infect new hosts to survive. Viruses that are able to travel between hosts successful have the ability to spread locally, nationally and internationally, causing a disease outbreak and ultimately a pandemic.

It is accepted that on the frontline in many countries, increasingly it is the nurses who screen, manage and support patients with suspected or confirmed COVID-19. These nurses often take microbiology and virology specimens and encounter infectious diseases in clinical practice. Therefore, it is essential that nurses understand the processes of disease transmission and disease prevention, but it is a cause for concern that a review of undergraduate nursing curricula revealed that microbiology and virology teaching are limited [3]. Recognizing that this situation is unlikely to change in the near future, it is essential that their gap in education is addressed. They need to gain the knowledge and skills to identify and recognize the specific signs and symptoms of infectious diseases such as SARS-CoV-2. In consequence, this chapter describes the pathophysiology of viruses and the current understanding of SARS-CoV-2.

COVID-19: A Critical Care Textbook. https://doi.org/10.1016/B978-0-12-815377-2.00001-9

Introduction to virology

Virology is the study of viruses and viral diseases [4]. It is important to point out at this stage that viruses are not classed as living organisms because they require a living host to survive, and are unable to independently reproduce and maintain metabolic activities. They are unable to go through mitosis (cell division), but are able to gain entry into a cell and then change the cell deoxyribonucleic acid (DNA) or ribonucleic acid (RNA), which enables them to survive and reproduce [4].

Viruses are extremely small, so to determine the shape and size of viral particles electron microscopy is used. Each virus has a unique shape that helps with identification and consists of one or two symmetrical shapes: icosahedral or helical shapes, with sizes varying from 20 to 300 nm in diameter [5]. The genome of viruses contains either DNA or RNA, with the capsid being a protein casing that surrounds the genome and the core proteins. Surrounding the capsid of some viruses is a lipid bilayer membrane referred to as an "envelope". This envelope contains glycoproteins with projections or spikes which allow the virus to attach firmly to the target cell. The process that transmits the infectious viral genome to the host cell is referred to as the "virion". As with all cells, it has to be noted that in some situations viral particles may lack nucleic acids or carry defective genomes, which limits normal cell replication [5].

All viruses need host cells to enable the synthesis of viral nucleic acids, proteins and progeny virions. Testing for viruses, laboratories culture the virus, and for diagnostic purposes use rapid molecular-based technology, such as polymerase chain reactions (PCRs) for DNA viruses and reverse-transcription PCR (RT-PCR) for RNA viruses [5].

After entering a host, replication of the virus within host cells entails six stages (Fig. 1.1). Firstly, the viral capsid (non-enveloped or enveloped) attaches to the cell surface receptor sites (Table 1.1). This causes an interaction between the viral glycoproteins and the host-cell surface, resulting in the virus then penetrating the host cell. This is followed by uncoating, the process through which the viral protein coat is removed allowing enzymes to release nucleic acid, and attach to the core proteins. The fourth stage involves the production of virus-specific mRNA, which forces the host's cell ribosome to alter to provide viral proteins (core, capsid). Morphogenesis and maturation then occur, leading to the production of subviral and viral particles. The final stage is the release of the virus by lysis (the bursting of infected cells) or by budding through the plasma membrane. It has to be noted that lysis causes cell death, whereas budding may not kill the cell, instead allowing viral particle shedding to continue. An example of budding is the hepatitis B infection, where the virus remains in the host cells and continues to release viral particles and antigens at a slow rate [5].

It is important to note that, in the latent infection phase, the virus does not undergo replication and viral nucleic acid remains within the host-cell cytoplasm, or becomes incorporated into the host genome [e.g., human immunodeficiency

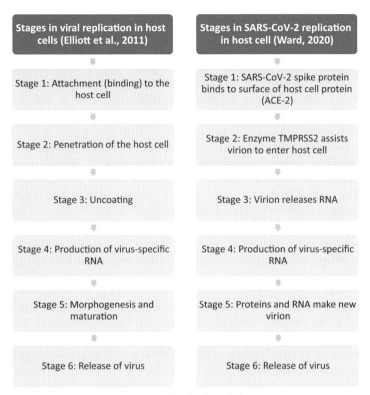

FIGURE 1.1   Replication of viruses.

TABLE 1.1 Non-enveloped and enveloped viruses [5]

Types	Examples
Non-enveloped viruses	Gastroenteritis, e.g., norovirus
Enveloped viruses	Influenza Chickenpox Herpes simplex virus Ebola

virus (HIV)]. When activated, viral replication, transcription and translation occur. Therapeutic options to control viral infections include blocking viral entry or replication using antiretroviral drugs or developing immunity for the uninfected population via vaccination [5,6].

Viruses require an incubation period from the time the host becomes infected to the onset of illness. Classification of transmission delineates whether the virus circulates within single species, for example, humans, or is able to cross the species barrier, transferring from animals to humans (zoonotic) and vice versa [7]. Viruses are transmitted person-to-person by horizontal or vertical routes. The horizontal route includes respiratory droplets, aerosol production, for example, coughing and sneezing, and gastrointestinal. The vertical route includes mother-to-child transmission, placental–foetal, or at delivery, for example, herpes simplex virus [5]. They are further classified according to the disease or organ system involved, virus family (nucleic acid type/virion structure), and the replication process [5].

The body has several natural defence mechanisms to prevent or contain infection. These include the epithelial surfaces of the body which are designed to prevent the infection entering the body. If the virus bypasses these barriers and initiates infection of a cell, then the host immune system is activated. A coordinated response of white blood cells, proteins and receptors attempts to control the infection, and provides long-term immunity, or resistance against the virus. The two main arms of the immune system, the innate immune system and adaptive immune system, overlap and coordinate the immune response [4].

The innate immune system is activated immediately, as is the non-specific response involving macrophages, dendritic cells, natural killer cells and innate cytokines (type 1 interferon) triggering the adaptive immune system. The adaptive immune system provides an antigen-specific response and consists of two major types of cells, T lymphocytes (T cells), and B lymphocytes (B cells). These cells are located within the lymph nodes and spleen, where the dendritic cells release the antigen to the T cells. T cells are deemed more important in the defence against viruses as they include cytotoxic T lymphocytes (CTLs) and helper T lymphocytes. CTLs destroy virally infected cells via apoptosis, and helper T cells activate other cell types, particularly B cells [4].

Coronaviruses in general

The first instance of coronavirus disease (HCoV-229E) in humans was found in the 1930s and isolated in 1965 [8]. These viruses (CoV) belong to the subfamily of *Orthocoronavirinae* in the family of Coronaviridae, order Nidovirales. There are four subtypes: Alphacoronavirus (α-CoV), Betacoronavirus (β-CoV), Gammacoronavirus (γ-CoV), and Deltacoronavirus (δ-CoV) [9,10]. Coronaviridae are complex, enveloped, positive-sense, single-stranded RNA viruses, between 60 and 220 nm in diameter. On an electron microscope, CoV are generally spherical, with large (approximately 20 nm) club- or petal-shaped proteins protruding on the cell surface; these are termed spikes (Picture 1.1). These protrusions give an image of a solar halo effect around the virus, like a crown (hence the designation corona) [7,12,13]. They are the means through which CoV are able to bind to receptors on the host cells, which in turn allows the release of viral RNA into the cell.

CoVs have been identified in humans (HCoV-NL63, HCoVOC43 and HCoV-HKU1) since the start of the 21st century, but until recently they were

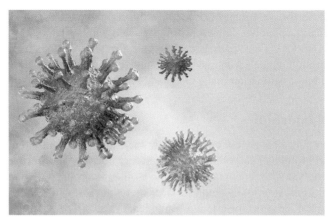

PICTURE 1.1   SARS-CoV-2 virus [11].

regarded as causing mild, self-limiting infections, such as the common cold. These viruses were estimated to cause 15–30% of respiratory tract infections annually [7,14]. However, severe acute respiratory syndrome (SARS; SARS-CoV), which transferred to humans from bats, marked a change in virulence, with increased severity of symptoms and mortality. Similarly, the Middle Eastern respiratory syndrome (MERS; MERS-CoV), identified in 2012, was linked to camels, and also caused severe respiratory diseases. In the more recent outbreaks of SARS and MERS, the viruses appear to have become more virulent and increasingly contagious [7,15].

SARS-CoV-2

SARS-CoV-2 belongs to the β coronavirus cluster [12,15] and is the third-identified zoonotic coronavirus disease. The genetic sequence of COVID-19 identified 80% similarity to SARS-CoV and 50% to MERS-CoV [16,17]. Thus, it is hypothesized that given the similar strain to that found in bats and humans, this is the route of transmission, however, its definitive origin remains unconfirmed [7,12,15,18].

The stages of replication (Fig. 1.1) are similar to those in other viruses. SARS-CoV-2 requires two key proteins, ACE2 is a receptor protein that allows the virus to dock to the host and TMPRRS2 that activates viral entry into the cell [19]. It binds to the transmembrane receptor ACE2, which is widely found in lung, heart, kidney, and gastrointestinal tissues [13]. Once the receptor binds the cell to access it, cleavage of the S protein (activated by the enzyme TMPRRS2) assists the virion to enter the cell which releases RNA. S proteins are divided into S1 and S2 categories, each of which has its own distinct function. S1 is responsible for receptor binding and S2 for cell membrane fusion. Once SARS-CoV-2 enters the cells it encounters the innate immune response. To effectively infect the host, the virus must be able to inhibit or evade host innate immune signalling. How this occurs remains unknown, however, it may have a similar pathogenesis mechanism to SARS-CoV. Once pathogenesis has occurred RNA is then translated into proteins through the cell machinery, with some replicated RNA. These are then assembled into a new virion in the Golgi and released [13,20].

Route of infection

SARS-CoV-2 is a highly contagious respiratory illness, currently thought to be transmitted through close contact and respiratory droplets of differing sizes and through direct or indirect contact with mucous membranes in the eyes, mouth or nose. The larger particles settle on surfaces more quickly, with smaller particles able to remain airborne for a longer time, leading to different modes of transmission [13]. It has been found that as the virus can survive on surfaces, infection can be either through inhalation and/or physical contact with the larger viral particles. Hence, routes of infection are multifaceted. In relatively closed environments and with continuous exposure to high concentrations of exhalations, aerosol generation of infection is possible [12,21]. When caring for COVID-19 patients, this route of infection has to be a cause for concern, because nursing and medical interventions include aerosol-generating procedures (AGPs) [22]. Examples of AGPs include humidification, open suctioning, non-invasive ventilation and intubation. The highest risk of transmission of respiratory viruses is during AGPs of the respiratory tract [22]. Following identification by Li et al. [23] that there was a lower risk of transmission when using Hudson, Venturi masks and nasal cannulae, as compared with high-flow nasal oxygen (HFNO) and non-invasive ventilation (NIV) with facemasks or hoods; these are now being used.

Inhalation of droplets results in the large particles contaminating the upper airways, with smaller particles (<5 μm) able to move into the lower respiratory tract. CoV-SARS-2 can also be spread from hand contact with viral particles on contaminated surfaces, for example, handrails, and then touching mucous membranes of the face (eyes, mouth and nose). It has been detected in faeces and urine, therefore this route of transmission is also possible [21].

Transmission

The rate of transmission of infection is described by the use of the reproductive (R) number calculation [12,13]. The R number used in public health is the estimated average number of infections generated by one infectious person in the population without immunity. In SARS-CoV-2, an additional challenge is that a number of individuals remain asymptomatic, making accurate calculation difficult [11]. Current thinking is that an R_0 of under 1 is necessary for infection to be seen as relatively low risk. As the R_0 number rises the infection risk to the population rises. It has to be noted that it is not unusual for R_0 estimates to vary, depending on the model and data used to calculate it [24] (see Chapter 3, p. 13).

The incubation period remains unclear, with most estimates ranging from 1 to 14 days, with an average 5 days before symptoms [21,25]. COVID-19 has both systemic and respiratory effects (Fig. 1.2), with an associated incidence among individuals with underlying diabetes, hypertension and cardiovascular disease [26]. Severe COVID-19 disease causes an aggressive pulmonary impact resulting in respiratory failure, similar to that of other viral pneumonias that cause respiratory failure [18]. However, due to its highly contagious nature, the risk of transmission is significant. It has to be accepted that in spontaneous self-ventilating patients, all oxygen administration strategies are at risk of aerosolization, which in turn increases risks for transmission [22].

Detection

Screening for SARS-Cov-2 involves a high nasopharyngeal and oropharyngeal swab based on an RT-PCR. RT-PCR is a molecular biological diagnosis technique based on nucleic acid sequence or by viral gene sequencing in swabs. A limitation to RT-PCR is that although it can confirm the presence of viral RNA it cannot provide information on the presence of infectivity, detection of prior infection or immunity for future infection [13]. In addition, accurate screening for COVID-19 is difficult as many individuals may be asymptomatic and, in consequence, are unlikely to be screened. There is also a possibility of false-negative results as screening is a one-point intervention, with a time delay to

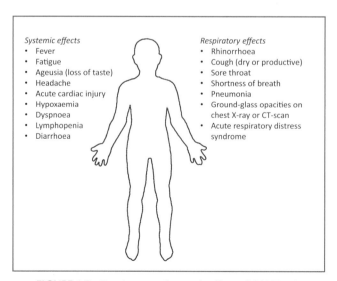

FIGURE 1.2 Respiratory and systemic effects of COVID-19.

results. This can mean that screened individuals may become infected post-screening but prior to results [27]. The procedure used for screening involves taking a high nasal swab, but this may lead to discomfort and bleeding, causing the professional to take an incomplete specimen.

A second form of screening, antibody testing, involves detection of an immune response to COVID-19, and its aim is to identify individuals who have been exposed and infected, and ascertain their resulting degree of immunity. In COVID-19 there are two issues with this form of screening. Firstly, antibody testing is not appropriate for acute diagnosis as it may take up to 7–10 days to seroconvert; in addition, current assays are only able to detect antibodies and not the evidence of immunity [13]. Secondly, recent evidence indicates that not all infected individuals generate sustained antibody responses [28]. However, from an epidemiological perspective this provides a greater understanding of the spread of infection and potentially identifies those with asymptomatic infections.

Summary

In recent years, global connectivity has led to an increase in the frequency of infections and potential pandemics. COVID-19 is the latest in the series of pandemics affecting human populations. Prior to 2020, it was over 100 years ago that a similar respiratory virus was recognized as infecting an estimated 500 million, with a morality of over 100 million people. CoV are highly vulnerable to public-health intervention strategies, and with the absence of a vaccine, the only effective intervention is to interrupt the transmission of virus through public-health prevention and control methods such as isolation and controlling the source of infection [12]. It is essential that nurses understand the virology of SARS-CoV-2, the route of infection, transmission and detection. Only then can the nurse use knowledge to prevent the spread of infection between patients and staff and provide effective evidence-based care.

References

[1] Hui DSEIA, Madani TA, Ntoumi F, Kock R, Dar O, et al. The containing of 2019-nCoV epidemic threat of novel coronaviruses in global health – the latest 2019 novel coronavirus outbreak in Wuhan, China. Int J Infect Dis 2020;91:264–6.

[2] World Health Organization. Naming the coronavirus disease (COVID-19) and the virus that causes it. 2020. Available from: https://www.who.int/emergencies/diseases/novel-coronavirus-2019/technical-guidance/naming-the-coronavirus-disease-%28covid-2019%29-and-the-virus-that-causes-it.

[3] Durrant R, Fenn JP. Microbiology education in nursing practice. J Microbiol Biol Educ 2017;18(2):1–8.

[4] Louten J. Essential human virology. Elsevier; 2016.

[5] Elliott T, Casey A, Sandoe J, Lambert A. Microbiology education in nursing practice. In: Lecture notes: medical microbiology and infection: medical microbiology and infection. John Wiley & Sons; 2011.

[6] Vardhana SA, Wolchock JD. The many faces of the anti-Covid immune response. J Exp Med 2020;217(6). E202000678.

[7] Weston D. Fundamentals of infection prevention and control: theory and practice. Wiley Blackwell; 2013.

[8] Kahn J, McIntosh K. History and recent advances in coronavirus discovery. Pediatr Infect Dis J 2005;24:s223–7.

[9] Banerjee A, Kulcsar K, Misra V, Frieman M, Mossman K. Bats and coronaviruses. Viruses 2019;11. https://doi.org/10.3390/v11010041. pii: E41.

[10] Yang D, Leibowitz JL. The structure and functions of coronavirus genomic 3′ and 5′ ends. Virus Res 2015;206:120–33. https://doi.org/10.1016/j.virusres.2015.02.025.

[11] Gov.uk. Coronavirus (COVID-19): scientific evidence supporting the UK government response. 2020. Available from: https://www.gov.uk/government/news/coronavirus-covid-19-scientific-evidence-supporting-the-uk-government-response.

[12] Li H, Liu SM, Yu XH, Tang SL, Tang CK. Coronavirus disease 2019 (COVID-19): current status and future perspectives. Int J Antimicrob Agents 2020:1–12. https://doi.org/10.1007/s42399-020-00619-z.

[13] Ward P. COVID-19/SARS-CoV-2 pandemic. In: Faculty of pharmaceutical medicine blog. 2020. Available from: https://www.fpm.org.uk/blog/covid-19-sars-cov-2-pandemic/.

[14] Coperchini F, Chiovato L, Croce L, Magri F, Rotondi M. The cytokine storm in COVID-19: an overview of the involvement of the chemokine/chemokine-receptor system. Cytokine Growth Factor Rev 2020;53:25–32.

[15] Sun P, Lu X, Xu C, Sun W, Pan B. Understanding of COVID−19 based on current evidence. J Med Virol 2020;92(6):548–551. https://doi.org/10.1002/jmv.25722.

[16] Ren LL, Wang YM, Wu ZQ, Xiang ZC, Guo L, Xu T, et al. Identification of a novel corona virus causing severe pneumonia in human: a descriptive study. Chinese Med J 2020;5(13.8):1015–1024. https://doi.org/10.1097/CM9.0000000000000722.

[17] Lu R, Zhao X, Li J, Niu P, Yang B, Wu H, et al. Genomic characterisation and epidemiology of 2019 novel coronavirus: implications for virus origins and receptor binding. Lancet 2020;395(10224):565–74. https://doi.org/10.1016/S01406736(20)30251-8.

[18] Park SE. Epidemiology, virology, and clinical features of severe acute respiratory syndrome -coronavirus-2 (SARS-CoV-2; Coronavirus Disease-19). CEP 2020;63(4):119–24. https://doi.org/10.3345/cep.2020.00493.

[19] Wighton S. Coronavirus 'map' identifies key virus entry points into the body. 2020. Available from: https://www.imperial.ac.uk/news/197114/coronavirus-identifies-virus-entry-points-into/.

[20] Harapan H, Itoh N, Yufika A, Winardi W, Keam S, Te H, et al. Coronavirus disease 2019 (COVID-19): a literature review. J Infect Public Health 2020;13(5):667–73.

[21] Public Health England. Guidance: Covid-19: epidemiology, virology and clinical features. 2020. Available from: https://www.gov.uk/government/publications/wuhan-novel-coronavirus-background-information/wuhan-novel-coronavirus-epidemiology-virology-and-clinical-features.

[22] Public Health England. COVID-19 infection prevention and control guidance: aerosol generating procedures. 2020. Available from: https://www.gov.uk/government/publications/wuhan-novel-coronavirus-infection-prevention-and-control/covid-19-infection-prevention-and-control-guidance-aerosol-generating-procedures.

[23] Li Y, Huang X, Yu IT, Wong TW, Qian H. Role of air distribution in SARS transmission during the largest nosocomial outbreak in Hong Kong. Indoor Air 2005;15:83–95.

[24] Coggan D, Rose G, Barker DJP. Chapter 1: what is epidemiology. In: Epidemiology for the uninhabited. 2020. Available from: www.bmj.com.

[25] Parasher A. COVID-19: current understanding of its pathophysiology, clinical presentation and treatment. Postgrad Med 2020. https://doi.org/10.1136/postgradmedj-2020-138577.

[26] Huang C, Wang Y, Li X, Ren L, Zhao J, Hu Y, et al. Clinical features of patients infected with 2019 novel coronavirus in Wuhan, China. Lancet 2020;395(10223):497–506. https://doi.org/10.1016/S0140-6736(20)30183-5.

[27] Kucirka LM, Lauer SA, Laeyendecker O. Variation in false-negative rate of reverse transcriptase polymerase chain reaction–based SARS-CoV-2 tests by time since exposure. Ann Intern Med 2020;173(4):262–267. https://doi.org/10.7326/M20-1495.

[28] World Health Organisation. "Immunity passports" in the context of COVID-19. 2020. Available from: https://www.who.int/news-room/commentaries/detail/immunity-passports-in-the-context-of-covid-19.

Chapter 2

Public health emergencies

Joy Notter, Chris Carter

Chapter Outline

Introduction

The recent COVID-19 pandemic has highlighted the importance of public health as countries face the impact of this latest public health emergency, and work to contain and prevent the spread of the virus. The internationally accepted definition of public health was first formulated by Acheson (1988) [1], and states that it is "the art and science of preventing disease, prolonging life and promoting health through the organized efforts of society" [1,2]. This definition clearly places the responsibility on countries to develop policies, health service structures, hospital and community programmes to increase and strengthen their national/public health capacity to protect and safeguard their communities. Traditionally public health has been divided into three areas, each of which has its own specific role in protecting the population. They are:

- Prevention: reducing the incidence of ill health, and supporting programmes for behaviour change to a healthier lifestyle
- Protection: the surveillance and monitoring of communicable diseases, emergency responses and immunization/vaccination programmes
- Promotion: the development and delivery of health education information and programmes, together with the commissioning of services designed to meet specific/targeted health needs.

Although the principles are internationally accepted, to be effective, public health provisions have to be tailored to fit within the cultural context of each country. Public health needs to focus on the entire spectrum of health and

COVID-19: A Critical Care Textbook. https://doi.org/10.1016/B978-0-12-815377-2.00001-9

well-being, not just the prevention and eradication of specific diseases. Services need to be designed with the aim of affording health services and conditions under which people take responsibility for their own health, accessing activities which promote health and well-being, or prevent deterioration of health.

Communicable diseases are infectious diseases caused by bacteria, viruses, parasites or fungi, spread directly or indirectly from one person to another. In public health terms, communicable diseases are referred to as endemic if they are constantly present in a country, with a similar or steady rate of infection among a population, for example, tuberculosis. The term outbreak is used when the incidence of the disease rises rapidly to well above the usual rate of infection, and epidemic is used when a specific health concern has spread to a larger geographical area. When spread across countries, or as in the case of COVID-19 across the world, the term pandemic is used. The term public health emergency is used when, as with a natural disaster, the impact of the spread of disease seriously disrupts the normal functioning of a community or a society, leading to widespread human, material, economic or environmental losses, exceeding the ability of the affected community or society to cope [2].

In recent years, public health emergencies from communicable diseases have included the Ebola virus outbreak in West Africa (2014–2015), the emergence of Zika virus (2015–2016), and yellow fever (2016) and cholera outbreaks (2018) in Africa [3]. The latest pandemic has revealed just how fragile the health systems are in many countries, forcing governments and service providers into making difficult choices on how to respond to try to meet the needs of their populations [4]. There are some excellent examples of countries whose public health responses have protected their communities, reducing the incidence and death rates from COVID-19. These countries, which include Vietnam (see Chapter 5), Australia, New Zealand, and South Korea (to cite just a few), rapidly deployed national strategies to contain and control spread of the virus, which included regulations governing public and social behaviour. An additional challenge is that public health emergencies are becoming more complex, as the rapidly evolving and advancing technology and communication lead to people, vectors and goods being continually moved not just across countries, but continents and worldwide (World Health Organization, 2020). International movement and travel, by acting as vectors to spread disease, pose an additional threat to the health of communities. In recognition of this, increasingly, there are major international public health responses to outbreaks of infectious diseases, with the World Health Organization (WHO) offering advice and guidance. They argue the importance of reducing travel and social contacts, with information developed regarding partial and total cessation of contact (lockdown), reduction of travel and quarantine measures, ways to protect individuals, care for vulnerable groups and communities, and the use of personal protection equipment (PPE).

It has to be noted that the terms public health emergency, disaster and major incident may be used interchangeably and mean different things to different people and organizations. Therefore, these terms will be defined in accordance with agreed international definitions. A public health emergency of international concern is defined by the WHO as

an extraordinary event which is determined to constitute a public health risk to other States through the international spread of disease and to potentially require a coordinated international response". This definition implies a situation that is serious, sudden, unusual or unexpected; carries implications for public health beyond the affected State's national border; and may require immediate international action [2].

Effective public health and social measures (PHSMs) to emergencies need to be based on local, national and international epidemiological information regarding how often and why a disease occurs in different groups and how a disease spreads [5]. Recognition and understanding of how plans and strategies are used have affected the spread and impact of the disease, can be used to develop new initiatives and strategies to improve protection of the population and support patients. PHSMs include personal protective measures (such as hand hygiene, respiratory etiquette and mask wearing); environmental measures (such as cleaning, disinfection and ventilation); surveillance and response measures (including contact tracing, isolation and quarantine); physical distancing measures (e.g., limiting the size of gatherings, maintaining distance in public or workplaces, domestic movement restrictions); and international travel-related measures [6]. PHSMs act in combination, with the implementation of a range of measures necessary for control to be effective. Measures used should be tailored to the lowest administrative level for which situational assessment is possible and measures can be enacted practically [6]. Internationally, there is an accepted range of terms and measures used in measuring disease outcomes in relation to the population at risk (PAR) that needs to be explored. The starting point has to be consideration of the chain of infection, using this strategies can be developed to intervene at key points and interrupt the cycle of events (Fig. 2.1), which unchecked lead to situations such as the current pandemic.

Internationally agreed definitions of terms are used, enabling local, national and international public health teams to share information and work together (Fig. 2.2).

When trying to assess the rate at which an infectious disease is spreading, epidemiologists calculate the reproduction rate of the disease, referred to as the "R" level. This is a mathematical term, and R_0, pronounced "R naught," indicates how contagious an infectious disease is by calculating the average number of people who will contract a contagious disease from one person with that disease. It is based on the assumption that the population of people were previously free of the infection, have no acquired immunity, and have not been vaccinated. COVID-19 is a new virus, so no one in the international population had had the disease, and vaccines did not exist. Using this measure, three possibilities exist (Fig. 2.3):

Firstly, the **infectious period**, the longer the infectious period of a disease, the more likely a person who has it can transmit the disease to other people. Therefore, a long period of infectiousness will contribute to a higher R_0 value.

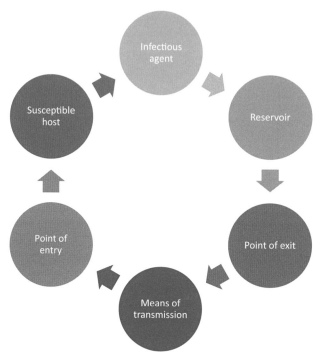

FIGURE 2.1 Chain of infection.

In common with most infections, there is an incubation period, a delay between the moment a person first becomes infected with COVID-19 and the appearance of the first symptoms. Currently, evidence suggests that the infection can be detected in people 1–3 days before their symptom onset, with the highest viral loads, as measured by RT-PCR, observed around the day of symptom onset, followed by a gradual decline over time [8–10]. The duration of RT-PCR positivity generally appears to be 1–2 weeks for asymptomatic persons, and up to 3 weeks or more for patients with mild-to-moderate disease [9,10]. In patients with severe COVID-19 disease, it can be much longer [8]. Secondly, the mode of transmission. The main aim of public health is to control COVID-19 by suppressing transmission of the virus and preventing associated illness and death. For this, a good understanding of the categories and modes of transmission is needed (Fig. 2.4).

Transmission of COVID-19 can occur through direct, indirect or close contact with infected people. Infected secretions, such as saliva and respiratory secretions or their respiratory droplets, are expelled through coughs, sneezes, speaking or singing [11,12]. Respiratory droplets are >5–10 μm in diameter, whereas droplets <5 μm in diameter are referred to as droplet nuclei or aerosols [13]. Respiratory droplet transmission can occur when a person is in close contact (within 1 m) with an infected person who has respiratory symptoms (e.g., coughing or sneezing) or who is talking or singing. Infected respiratory droplets can reach the mouth, nose or eyes of a susceptible person, transmitting the infection. Indirect contact

Term	Definition
Suspected case	A person with acute respiratory illness (fever and at least one sign/symptom of respiratory disease, e.g., cough, sore throat, headache, fatigue, shortness of breath), AND a history of travel to or residence in a country/area or territory reporting local transmission of COVID-19 during the 14 days prior to symptom onset **Or** A person with any acute respiratory illness AND having been in contact with a confirmed or probable COVID-19 case in the last 14 days prior to symptom onset **Or** A person with severe acute respiratory illness (fever and at least one sign/symptom of respiratory disease, e.g., cough, sore throat, headache, fatigue, shortness of breath), AND requiring hospitalization AND in the absence of an alternative diagnosis that fully explains the clinical presentation
Probable case	A suspect case for whom testing for COVID-19 is inconclusive or who tested positive using a pan-corona virus assay AND without laboratory evidence of other respiratory pathogens **Or** Any suspect case or death with an epidemiological link to a confirmed case(s) **Or** Any suspect case with typical COVID-19 appearance in chest computed tomography (CT scan) or chest X-ray
Confirmed COVID-19 Death	A person with laboratory confirmation of COVID-19 infection, irrespective of clinical signs and symptoms
Suspected COVID-19 Death	A death resulting from an illness that is clinically compatible with suspected or probable COVID-19 illness, OR a death where there is no clear alternative cause (e.g., trauma)

FIGURE 2.2 COVID-19 case definitions [7].

R value	Meaning
R_0 is less than 1 (<1)	Each person who is infected, passes the infection on to less than one new infection In this case, the disease will decline and eventually die out
R_0 equals 1	Each person who is infected causes one new infection The disease will stay alive and stable, but there will not be an outbreak or epidemic
R_0 is more than 1 (>1)	Each person who is infected causes more than one new infection The disease will be transmitted between people, and there may be an outbreak or epidemic

FIGURE 2.3   R levels.

transmission involving contact of a susceptible host with a contaminated object or surface (fomite transmission) may also be possible.

Airborne transmission of COVID-19 is also possible. This is when infected droplet nuclei (aerosols) remain infectious while suspended in air over long distances and time [13]. This can occur naturally following coughing, or during medical procedures that generate aerosols (aerosol-generating procedures) [3]. Thus, a susceptible person could inhale aerosols and become infected. Although the proportion of exhaled droplet nuclei or respiratory droplets that evaporate to generate aerosols required to cause infection in another person is not currently known, this route has been studied in other respiratory viruses and all precautions including PPE must be used with COVID-19 patients [14].

Currently, evidence is emerging that transmission from asymptomatic individuals may occur [15]. However, it is important to distinguish between transmission from people who are infected who never develop symptoms [15] (asymptomatic transmission) and transmission from people who are infected but have not developed symptoms yet (presymptomatic transmission). Multiple studies have shown that people infect others before they themselves became ill [12,16,17], but the extent of truly asymptomatic infection in the community remains unknown. The proportion of people whose infection is asymptomatic likely varies, but studies do indicate that children are less likely to show clinical symptoms compared to adults [18].

Fomite transmission is when respiratory secretions or droplets expelled by infected individuals contaminate surfaces and objects, creating fomites

Transmission classification	Definitions [3] *Countries, territories or areas with:*
No (active) cases	No cases or no new cases detected for at least 28 days (two times the maximum incubation period for COVID-19), in the presence of an effective surveillance system. This implies a near-zero risk of infection for the general population
Imported/ sporadic cases	Cases detected in the past 14 days are all imported, sporadic (e.g., laboratory acquired or zoonotic) or are all linked to imported/sporadic cases, and there are no clear signals of further locally acquired transmission. This implies minimal risk of infection for the general population
Cluster of cases	Cases detected in the past 14 days are predominantly limited to well-defined clusters that are not directly linked to imported cases, but which are all linked by time, geographic location **and** common exposures. It is assumed that there are a number of unidentified cases in the area. This implies a low risk of infection to others in the wider community if exposure to these clusters is avoided
Community transmission levels	**Level 1 (CT1)**: **Low incidence** of locally acquired, widely dispersed cases detected in the past 14 days, with many of the cases not linked to specific clusters; transmission may be focused in certain population sub-groups. Low risk of infection for the general population **Level 2 (CT2)**: **Moderate incidence** of locally acquired, widely dispersed cases detected in the past 14 days; transmission less focused in certain population sub-groups. Moderate risk of infection for the general population **Level 3 (CT3)**: **High incidence** of locally acquired, widely dispersed cases in the past 14 days; transmission widespread and not focused in population sub-groups. High risk of infection for the general population **Level 4 (CT4)**: **High incidence** of locally acquired, widely dispersed cases in the past 14 days; transmission widespread and not focused in population sub-groups. High risk of infection for the general population

FIGURE 2.4   Transmission information.

(contaminated surfaces). Viable COVID-19 virus and/or RNA detected by RT-PCR can be found on those surfaces for periods ranging from hours to days, depending on the ambient environment (including temperature and humidity) and the type of surface, in particular at high concentration in healthcare facilities where COVID-19 patients were being treated [19–22]. Therefore, transmission may also occur indirectly through touching surfaces in the immediate environment or objects contaminated with virus from an infected person (e.g., a stethoscope or thermometer), followed by touching the mouth, nose or eyes. Fomite transmission is considered a likely mode of transmission for SARS-CoV-2, given consistent findings about environmental contamination in the vicinity of infected cases and the fact that other coronaviruses and respiratory viruses can transmit this way.

Other modes of transmission of concern for all healthcare professionals include that COVID-19 (SARS-CoV-2) RNA has also been detected in biological samples, including urine, faeces [8,23], and in plasma or serum, and it is known that the virus can replicate itself in blood cells. However, the role of blood borne transmission remains uncertain; and low viral load in plasma and serum suggest that the risk of transmission through this route may be low [24]. This emerging evidence, although not yet corroborated by research demonstrating transmission through these media, confirms the need for nurses caring for critically ill COVID-19 patients to be scrupulously careful when handling any and all bodily fluids from patients.

Thirdly, the contact rate, this refers to the number of persons the infected individual has had contact with. If a person with a contagious disease comes into contact with many people who are not infected or vaccinated, the disease will be transmitted more quickly. However, if that person remains at home, in a hospital, or otherwise quarantined while they are contagious, the disease will be transmitted more slowly. A high contact rate will contribute to a higher R_0 value, and evidence demonstrates that limiting close contact between infected people and others is central to breaking chains of transmission of the virus causing COVID-19. The prevention of transmission is best achieved by identifying suspect cases as quickly as possible, testing, and isolating infectious cases [25,26]. In addition, it is critical to identify all close contacts of infected people [25] and place them in quarantine to limit spread and reduce transmission [25]. By quarantining close contacts, potential secondary cases will already be separated from others before they develop symptoms or become infectious, if they are infected, further preventing the chances of onward spread.

In consequence, a key strategy in preventing the transmission between persons is contact tracing. A contact is an individual (or group of individuals) who was within two metres of a probable or confirmed case starting from 2 days before illness onset (or for asymptomatic cases 2 days prior to positive specimen connection) until the time the person is isolated. Contact tracing is defined as the identification and systematic follow-up of persons who meet the definition of a contact of an infectious disease such as COVID-19. Figure 2.5 is the

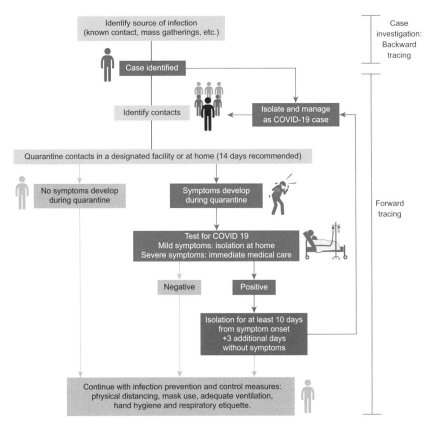

FIGURE 2.5 Chain of events for tracing, monitoring and caring for contacts of probable and confirmed COVID-19 cases.

WHO-developed process for contact tracing which has been adapted by many countries [5].

This shows the importance of using a system that is logical, and gives clear instructions of the steps to follow at each stage of the contact tracing process. Using a pictorial chart enables both staff and those being traced to follow the rationale behind the contact tracing process. In the hospital setting, a patient that presents in the emergency department will need to be referred to the relevant public health authority. In addition, hospitals will need to maintain records of numbers of patients seen and referred, and their outcomes. As part of this process the investigation team could follow the WHO [3] guide to key information needed (Fig. 2.6).

In many countries, legislation may be implemented to meet the new public health requirements as countries strive to contain the virus. For example, without social distancing, in normal social settings, an individual with COVID-19 can be expected to infect around three others over the course of their infection. One "generation" of infection takes around 1 week. So after 1 week, one infected individual will have become four infected individuals (the original

Type of Information	Minimum data required
Contact identification	• Contact (unique) ID • Linked source Case ID or Event ID • Full name • Address (and geolocation, where possible) • Phone number and/or other contact details • Alternative contact details (important in settings with variable telecommunications reception)
Demographic information	• Sex • Occupation (to identify healthcare workers, transport workers, other at-risk occupations) • Relationship with the source case • Language (in settings with diverse populations)
Type of contact	• Type of contact (household, workplace, community, health facility, other) • Date of last contact with the COVID-19 patient • Exposure frequency and duration (this may be used to classify contacts into high or low exposure in case resources are too limited to allow for tracing of all contacts) • Factors influencing contact vulnerability
Daily follow-up of signs and symptoms	• **Fever** (perceived or measured, and reported or observed) • **Other signs and symptoms:** sore throat, cough, runny nose or nasal congestion, shortness of breath or difficulty breathing, muscle pain, loss of smell or taste, or diarrhoea
Absence of loss of contact	• Reasons for non-reporting of daily signs and symptoms (contacts are unavailable, relocated, lost to follow-up) • New address (if known)
Additional activities Take COVID-19 PVR test then communicate result of COVID-19 PCR test to contact Contact discontinues self-isolation after 14 days from last exposure if asymptomatic	

FIGURE 2.6   Contact information and data [42].

How infection in one person can be transmitted to others

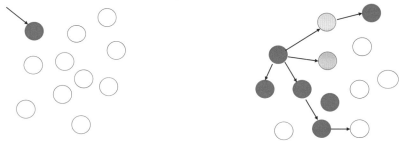

Adapted from Kingston
University London

Controlling Outbreaks: COVID-19 comparison numbers

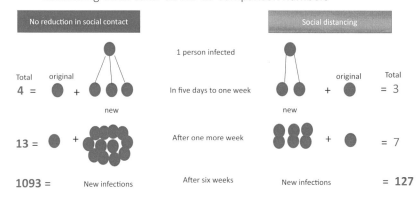

FIGURE 2.7   Illustration of differences in transmission with and without social distancing [27].

infected individual, plus the three individuals they have infected). After a further week, each of the three new infected individuals can be expected to cause three new infections, leading to 13 infections in total (Fig. 2.7). This compounding effect continues, so that after 6 weeks, as Thompson (2020) points out, the initial infected individual will have started a chain of transmission that has led to over 1000 infections [27].

Two other terms are quality-adjusted life years (QALYs) and disability-adjusted life years (DALYs). QALYs provide an agreed system for assessing the extent of the benefits gained from medical interventions/treatments in terms of health-related quality of life and survival for the patient. When combined with the costs of the interventions/treatments, cost–utility ratios result; these indicate the additional costs required to generate a year of perfect health (one QALY). Using this comparisons can be made between interventions, for clarity these have been called Intervention A and Intervention B, and priorities can be established based on those interventions that are relatively inexpensive (low

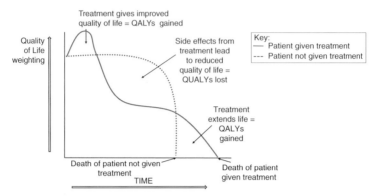

FIGURE 2.8 Comparison of the outcomes of treatment and non-treatment for a patient with a poor prognosis.

cost per QALY) and those that are relatively expensive (high cost per QALY). QALYs are worked out using the equation given:

$$\text{Cost-utility ratio} = \frac{\text{Cost of Intervention A} - \text{Costs of Intervention B}}{\substack{\text{No. of QALYs produced} \\ \text{by Intervention A}} - \substack{\text{No. of QALYs produced} \\ \text{by Intervention B}}}$$

Fig. 2.8 demonstrates how QALYs can be used to measure the differences in outcomes between treating and non-treating of a condition with a poor prognosis. The graph shows that treatment has an initial improvement on health-related quality of life, but as any adverse side-effects from treatment arise, their impact adversely affects the patient's quality of life. The result of this is that the benefits of treatment become lost, and the quality of life of the treated patient falls below that expected for a non-treated patient. This is described as a quality of life deficit, and referred to as "QALYs lost" when compared with a non-treated patient. The time of death of a non-treated patient is then compared with that of a treated patient. Fig. 2.8 shows that the treated patient lives longer, so demonstrates "QALYs gained" by virtue of their continued life, although as the graph shows at a lower quality of life. In medicine and nursing, one of the major dilemmas is deciding between a longer survival time with a reduced health-related quality of life and a shorter survival time with a better health-related quality of life. In a pandemic such as COVID-19, with its rapid deterioration and life-threatening complications, making this decision becomes only too common. Staff may well need psychological support to cope with this ongoing stressful and distressing circumstance.

It is being increasingly recognized that with COVID-19, recovery from the virus, the rapid deterioration in health status, and accompanying complications experienced has led to high-intensity treatments given in critical care, which come at a high cost for all countries. Therefore, it is likely that the full cost,

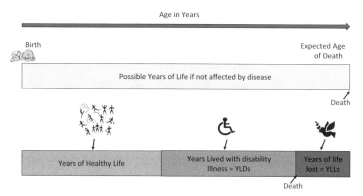

FIGURE 2.9 Illustration of components of DALYs.

using this definition, will only be calculated after the pandemic lessens its hold, and healthcare services can try to recover their prepandemic level. However, it is accepted that the long-term implications of these costs will adversely impact on service delivery possibilities for some years to come, particularly in low-/middle-income countries (LMICs), which at all times struggle to provide equitable services to their communities. The situation is compounded because an emerging complication of COVID-19 is long COVID [28]. This is when survivors of the pandemic are left with long-term symptoms and disabilities. For this group, physiotherapy and other treatments may be needed for a considerable time, and at this time it is unclear as to whether all patients will recover completely or not.

When quantifying the burden of a disease, long-term consequences/ongoing morbidity need to be recognized, and for this it may be appropriate to use the DALY. The DALY estimates how much the disease affects or burdens the life of the population. It is the primary metric used by the WHO to assess the global burden of disease (GBD). DALYs combine in one consistent, internationally recognized measure the burden from firstly, its mortality: years lost because of premature death due to disease; and secondly its morbidity: years of life lived adversely affected by disease (Fig. 2.9). Years of life lost as a result of premature death are compared to a standard life expectancy, this varies from country to country, with high-income countries (HICs) having a higher standard life expectancy than Low Middle Income Countries (LMICs) (for example in the UK it is usually 80 years for men and 82 years for women).

One DALY is the term used to represent the loss of the equivalent of one year of full health. YLL relates to the number of deaths multiplied by the standard life expectancy at the age death occurs. The calculation is as follows:

$$YLL = number\,(n) \times standard\ life\ expectancy\ at\ age\ of\ death\ in\ years\,(L)$$

YLDs refers to the years the patient lives with a disability, and represents an attempt to convert *years of life affected by a disability into the same terms as years of life lost due to premature death.* A numerical weighting is applied to each disease based on an accepted calculation as the impact that a particular disease has on life. Clear examples of internationally accepted weighting for diseases can be found in the GBD, the most comprehensive global epidemiological study [29] first published in 1990 this has been updated regularly. Thus, DALYs for a disease or health condition are the sum of the years of life lost due to premature mortality (YLLs) and the years lived with a disability (YLDs) arising after the disease or health condition, using the agreed weighting as to how much the disability affects health. Using these the DALY is calculated as follows:

$$DALY = YLL + YLD$$

This can give a national or international indication of the total burden of a disease, yet to be calculated for COVID-19, but likely to form an internationally accepted indicator of the burden of the disease on all nations, if as with many other viruses and diseases, it cannot be eradicated.

The role of the critical care nurse

New infectious diseases such as COVID-19 are a significant threat to global health and security. In extreme situations, such as a pandemic or outbreak, public health ethics take precedence. However, these may be less understood than the accepted professional values, principles and medical codes of ethics, integral elements of all undergraduate, postgraduate nurse education programmes, and clinical practice [30,31]. The overriding principles of public health ethics recognize the need to restrict individual choice in an effort to prevent, contain and/or promote health [32]. However, there is a fine line between medical and public health ethics, with a moral dilemma regarding the question of when the interests of the population override the rights of the individual, and whether decisions are based on political rather than health agendas. This is clearly evident in the tensions that arise when regulations are introduced to prevent the spread of an infectious disease, for example, forced quarantine, self-isolation and the challenges accompanying hospital admissions and treatment when services are in danger of becoming overwhelmed [32].

In the light of limited ethical and professional models designed for use in a pandemic, there is a need to draw guidance from other sources, such as national/international conflict and disaster emergencies, where there is a constant interplay between ethics, professional codes and morals [31]. As hospitals respond to a public health emergency such as a pandemic, they may utilize pre-prepared major incident plans, which may include action cards for key members of staff, to outline their responsibilities and roles. These have agreed sets of priorities which include command, safety, communication, assessment, triage, treatment and transport (CSCATTT) [33]. These need to be carefully reviewed and used to devise practical tools that critical care nurses can use to help them in their decision-making in the unprecedented situations they face daily.

The nature of infectious disease outbreaks such as SARS-CoV-2 result in critical care referrals increasing exponentially, with sharing of resources needed as organizations move nearer and nearer to the point of exhaustion of resources [34]. There is inevitably an accompanying need for extension in critical care nursing and medical capacity, greater ICU space, additional supplies, and medications. The situation becomes compounded when the nature of the disease means wards and critical care units have patients who need prolonged intensive care, which leads to an extended duration of admission. In consequence, planning needs to account not only for rapidly rising numbers that go well beyond normal provision, but also for extensive lengths of stay in critical care and high-dependency units [34].

During an infectious disease outbreak such as COVID-19, hospital and, in particular, critical care services face the risk of becoming overwhelmed, as each day dynamically evolves and changes. Pathways for suspected and confirmed infections and those who are negative need to be identified to prevent uncontrolled spread within units and wards. For many hospitals, emergency services and other essential services, for example, dialysis and cancer diagnosis and treatment, need to continue, with all attendance increasing possibilities for transmission to vulnerable groups, for example, those immunocompromised receiving chemotherapy. Staff, too, need to be protected and regularly tested, with vulnerable staff (including those who are pregnant), segregated from staff working in COVID-19 areas. One of the biggest problems is that staff who have been in contact with a colleague who tests positive then have to isolate for 14 days from other staff to prevent the risk of cross-contamination and transmission, which further reduces the overstretched workforce.

Recognition of the impact of the extreme circumstances arising from COVID-19 on critical care led to the COVID-19 Framework for critical care response given below [35,36]. This indicates three levels of response, and can be used as a guide as waves of the pandemic arise and recede (Fig. 2.10).

Transferring patients to other hospitals may be necessary to create capacity for new admissions. In the UK, during the COVID-19 pandemic between March and May 2020, the NHS established five emergency hospitals throughout England to treat 10,000 COVID-19 patients [37]. Although these units were not required, these large-scale critical care units aimed to decompress and reduce the pressure on hospitals. However, it has to be noted that during non-pandemic times, transferring critically ill patients has been shown to have an adverse event rate of 6.5%, with hypotension and haemodynamic instability and hypoxia [38]. During a pandemic, patients may not be adequately optimized prior to transfer and the transfer team may be junior or have limited experience of undertaking specialist critical care transfers. In consequence, the establishment of specialist transfer teams may be initiated to facilitate transfers within a given region.

COVID-19 demonstrates an unusual reversal of the usual trend of infectious disease impact on countries, with those most affected by COVID-19 and with most reported deaths being high-income countries [39]. This is a total change

	Normal	Surge	Extreme
Space	Usual patient care spaces maximized with overall bed occupancy below 85% COVID-19 suspected/positive and COVID-19-negative critical care bed and pathway separation assessed, agreed upon and enacted Enhanced areas for equipment and consumables identified and available Staff support, administration, rest and well-being facilities prepared	Enhanced areas for critical care identified and re-purposed, e.g., theatre recovery)	Non-traditional areas used for critical care areas, e.g., ward areas Critical care interventions being provided in non-critical care areas, e.g., NIV/CPAP being initiated in ward areas Requirement to transfer critically ill patients to other facilities to provide capacity
Staff	Baseline staffing levels compliant with national guidelines for all staff groups Additional critical care staff available Written record of areas of clinical competency for all unit staff and for the workforce supporting expanded and surge capacity Identification of roles and specific staff members who are to be allocated to critical care rotas to support expansion and surge capacity Well-being initiatives incorporated into baseline activity Ongoing permanent appointments made to existing vacancies as necessary	Trained critical care staff supervising larger number of patients, changes in responsibilities and documentation Well-being support programme described and information cascaded to all staff Staff members for expanded/surge workforce not identified	Sickness rates or staff who are required to 'shield' at or above 15% of established workforce Insufficient critical care trained staff available /unable to care for volume of patients, care team model increased with non-critical care trained staff Critical care staffing ratios significantly higher than pre-pandemic levels and reliant on non-ICU staff Insufficient downtime for recuperation after previous intense care episodes Staffing models for expanded/surge workforce not identified
Stuff	Sufficient flexible capacity of invasive and non-invasive ventilators to support surge patient numbers Secure stocks of commonly used medicines to support expanded bed numbers Full equipment inventory and plan for redeployment in event of expansion or surge Sufficient resources, consumables, drugs and re-supply available	Planned use of anaesthetic machines for short-term patient ventilation, with a view to using mechanical ventilators for patients requiring longer term ventilation Inadequate on-site stock of consumables for surge capacity Incomplete equipment inventory In consequence, conservation of supplies with selected re-use of supplies when safe	Critical shortage of supplies, drugs. Possible allocation/re-allocation of resources PPE shortages or inadequate or incomplete staff fit testing Inadequate on-site stock of consumables for expanded capacity Insufficient equipment identified for expanded bed space numbers
Systems	Normal systems function and able to adapt and respond to changing service needs	New management structures and work streams created in response to operational problems Organization able to cope with increased demand	Critical care overwhelmed. Not consistent with usual standard of care. Model is based on fundamental care and maintaining patient safety
Standard of Care	Usual care Able to increase bed-capacity by 20% with minimal effect on staff	100% increase in bed-capacity Changes in standard to care. Critical care nurse to patient ratio reduced Changes in nursing care model	200% increase in bed-capacity Triage and revised admission/discharge criteria introduced Patients needed to be transferred out to other hospitals

FIGURE 2.10   COVID-19 framework for critical care response [35,36].

in direction, previously HICs sought to protect themselves from infectious diseases from low- and low–middle-income countries that were considered to have high rates of neglected tropical diseases and outbreaks of infectious diseases. This reversal from HICs providing guidance and aid has revealed that well-resourced healthcare systems rapidly shifted their focus as they struggled to cope with the consequences of the COVID-19 pandemic. Critical care existing resources have been stretched well beyond normal usage, and as the pandemic continues, for staff there is an ongoing and unceasing demand which gives no time for rest and recovery. Instead as they continue to try to maintain service delivery, the risk of burn out and post-traumatic stress disorder (PTSD) rises exponentially. In addition, it has to be recognized that in the current climate, future service needs and the ability to respond remain unknown. Innovative approaches are needed to redress shortages and support the continuance of services, with lessons learned from peers in LMICs helping to facilitate altered usage of equipment and resources. There is another issue for critical care units, there is intense pressure to try to maintain normal service delivery, which brings its own challenges. As normal services are reduced, this in turn impacts on other patients, and it is estimated that there will be major increases in mortality from other causes, including untreated cancers. Also, in some instances, delays in surgery and medicine [40] will cause additional complications that will affect the time and level of care needed once routine procedures are resumed, further reducing the health of the community.

Conclusion

When initially reviewing critical care and the role of nurses, public health can seem remote from their everyday role. However, it is essential that all healthcare professionals follow national and international trends in health and illness and are able to work with their peers and managers to implement in a timely manner the strategies designed to protect them, their patients and the public. Unlike many diseases that have been known over time, COVID-19 reached pandemic status incredibly quickly, in public health terms it has demonstrated three defining characteristics: the disease spread globally rapidly and had an explosive spread and impact even on the world's most resilient health systems; the severity of cases; and finally the deep societal and economic disruption and consequences of the disease [41,42]. Protecting health workers who were risking their lives to fight the pandemic was and is one of WHO's biggest public health priorities. Infections escalated so rapidly that internationally there was an acute shortage of essential supplies, as health systems struggled to obtain the necessary PPE and other clinical equipment. At the same time other public health strategies had to be developed to protect the public at large and contain the spread of disease. The rapid transmission that can occur when social distancing is reduced, the difficulties of contact tracing and the high global death rate give indicators of just how difficult this is and the urgent need for all to follow public health guidelines to reduce and minimize further spread. For critical care nurses already exhausted by many months of working beyond normal capacity, strategies need to be developed to support them clinically and psychologically, or the additional risk is that they will be unable to continue in their vital role.

References

[1] Acheson ED. On the state of the public health [the fourth Duncan lecture]. Public Health 1988;102(5):431–7.

[2] World Health Organization. (2019). Emergencies: International health regulations and emergency committees. https://www.who.int/news-room/q-a-detail/emergencies-international-health-regulations-and-emergency-committees.

[3] World Health Organization. Communicating risk in public health emergencies. 2020.

[4] World Health Organization. A WHO guideline for emergency risk communication (ERC) policy and practice. 2020. https://www.who.int/risk-communication/guidance/download/en/.

[5] World Health Organisation. (2021). Contact tracing in the context of Covid-19. Interim guidance. 1st February 2021. www.who.int.

[6] World Health Organization. Taxonomy and glossary of public health and social measures that may be implemented to limit the spread of COVID-19. 2020. https://www.who.int/docs/default-source/documents/phsm/20200923-phms-who-int.zip?sfvrsn=691966ba_2.

[7] World Health Organisation. WHO Covid-19 case definition. 2020. https://www.who.int/publications/i/item/WHO-2019-nCoV-Surveillance_Case_Definition-2020.2.

[8] Pan Y, Zhang D, Yang P, Poon LLM, Wang Q. Viral load of SARS-CoV-2 in clinical samples. Lancet Infect Dis 2020;20(4):411–2.

[9] He, Lau EH, Wu P, Deng X, Wang J, Hao X, et al. Temporal dynamics in viral shedding and transmissibility of COVID-19. Nat Med 2020;26(5):672–5.

[10] Wölfel R, Corman VM, Guggemos W, Seilmaier M, Zange S, Müller MA, et al. Virological assessment of hospitalized patients with COVID-2019. Nature 2020;581(7809):465–9.

[11] Liu J, Liao X, Qian S, Yuan J, Wang F, Liu Y, et al. Community transmission of severe acute respiratory Syndrome Coronavirus 2, Shenzhen. Emerg Infect Dis 2020;26:1320–3.

[12] Luo L, Liu D, Liao X, Wu X, Jing Q, Zheng J, et al. Modes of contact and risk of transmission in COVID-19 among close contacts (pre-print). MedRxiv 2020. https://doi.org/10.1101/2020.03.24.20042606.

[13] World Health Organisation. Infection prevention and control of epidemic-and pandemic-prone acute respiratory infections in health care. 2014. www.who.int.

[14] Gralton J Tovey TR, McLaws M-L, Rawlinson WD. Respiratory Virus RNA is detectable in airborne and droplet particles. J Med Virol 2013;85:2151–9.

[15] World Health Organization. Considerations in the investigation of cases and clusters of COVID-19: interim guidance. 2020. www.who.int/publications/i/item/considerations-in-the-investigation-of-cases-and-clusters-of-covid-19.

[16] Yu P, Zhu J, Zhang Z, Han Y. A familial cluster of infection associated with the 2019 novel coronavirus indicating possible person-to-person transmission during the incubation period. J Infect Dis 2020;221(11):1757–61.

[17] Tong Z-D, Tang A, Li K-F, Li P, Wang H-L, Yi J-P, et al. Potential presymptomatic transmission of SARS-CoV-2, Zhejiang Province, China, 2020. Emerg Infect Dis 2020;26(5):1052–4.

[18] Davies N, Klepac P, Liu Y, Prem K, Jit M. Age-dependent effects in the transmission and control of COVID-19 epidemics. Nat Med 2020. https://doi.org/10.1038/s41591-020-0962-9.

[19] Van Doremalen N, Bushmaker T, Morris DH, Holbrook MG, Gamble A, Williamson BN, et al. Aerosol and surface stability of SARS-CoV-2 as compared with SARS-CoV-1. N Engl J Med 2020;382:1564–7.

[20] Chia PY, Coleman KK, Tan YK, Ong SWX, Gum M, et al. Detection of air and surface contamination by SARS-CoV-2 in hospital rooms of infected patients. Nat Commun 2020;11:1.

[21] Guo Z-D, Wang Z-Y, Zhang S-F, Li X, Li L, Li C, et al. Aerosol and surface distribution of severe acute respiratory syndrome coronavirus 2 in hospital wards, Wuhan, China. Emerg Infect Dis 2020;26:7.

[22] Zhou J, Otter J, Price JR, Cimpeanu C, Garcia DM, Kinross J, et al. Investigating SARS-CoV-2 surface and air contamination in an acute healthcare setting during the peak of the COVID-19 pandemic in London (pre-print). MedRxiv 2020. https://doi.org/10.1101/2020.05.24.20110346.

[23] Wang W, Xu Y, Gao R, Lu R, Han K, Wu G, et al. Detection of SARS-CoV-2 in different types of clinical specimens. J Am Med Assoc 2020;323(18):1843–4.

[24] Chang L, Zhao L, Gong H, Wang L, Wang L. Severe acute respiratory Syndrome Coronavirus 2 RNA detected in blood donations. Emerg Infect Dis 2020;26:1631–3.

[25] World Health Organisation. Considerations for quarantine of individuals in the context of containment for coronavirus disease (COVID-19): interim guidance. 2020. https://www.who.int/publications/i/item/considerations-for-quarantine-of-individuals-in-the-context-of-containment-for-coronavirus-disease-(covid-19.

[26] World Health Organisation. Global surveillance for COVID-19 caused by human infection with COVID-19 virus: interim guidance. 2020. www.who.int/publications/i/item/global-surveillance-for-covid-19-caused-by-human-infection-with-covid-19-virus-interim-guidance.

[27] Thompson R, Coronavirus modelling - why social distancing works Mathematical Institute, University of Oxford 2020 http//www.maths.oc.ac.uk/node/35371.

[28] National Institute for Health and Care Excellence. COVID-19 rapid guideline: managing the long-term effects of COVID-19. NICE Guideline 188; 2020. https://www.nice.org.uk/guidance/NG188.

[29] Lancet. The global burden of disease. 2021. https://www.thelancet.com/gbd.

[30] World Health Organisation. State of world nursing report. 2020. https://www.who.int/publications/i/item/9789240003279.

[31] International Council of Nurses. Code of ethics. 2012. www.icn.ch.

[32] Clay KA, Henning JD, Horne S. Op GRITROCK ethics; the way of things to come? J Roy Army Med Corps 2016;162(3):150–5.

[33] National Health Service England. Clinical guidelines for major incidents and mass casualty events. 2018. https://www.england.nhs.uk/wp-content/uploads/2018/12/version1__Major_Incident_and_Mass_casualty_guidelines-Nov-2018.pdf.

[34] Hossain T, Ghazipura M, Dichter JR. Intensive care role in disaster management in critical care clinics. Crit Care Clin 2019;35:535–50.

[35] Royal College of Anaesthetists. Restarting planned surgery in the context of the Covid-19 pandemic. 2020.

[36] Christian MD, Devereaux AV, Dichter JR. Introduction and executive summary: care of the critically ill and injured during the pandemics and disasters. CHEST Consens Statement 2014;146(Suppl. l):85–345.

[37] Day M. Covid-19: Nightingale hospitals set to shut down after seeing few patients. BMJ 2020;369. m1860.

[38] Singh JM, MacDonald RD, Ahghari M. Critical events during land-based inter facility transport. Ann Emerg Med 2014;64(1):9–15. E12.

[39] Cash R, Patel V. The art of medicine: had Covid-19 subverted global health? Lancet 2020;395:1687–8.

[40] Lancet Rheumatology. Too long to wait: the impact of COVID-19 on elective surgery. Lancet Rheumatology 2021;3:E83.

[41] Czeisler ME, Marynak K, Clarke KEN, Salah Z, Shakya I, Thierry JM, Ali N, McMilllan H, Wiley JF, et al. Delays or avoidance of medical care because of Covid-19 related concerns. United States, June 2020. In: Centre of disease control and prevention. ;69. 2020. p. 1250–7. Weekly, 36.

[42] Centres for Diseases. Contact tracing for Covid-19. 2020. https://www.cdc.gov/coronavirus/2019-ncov/php/contact-tracing/contact-tracing-plan/contact-tracing.html.

Chapter 3

Critical care nurse leadership

Chris Carter, Martine Rooney, Joy Notter

Chapter Outline

The unprecedented demand for critical care services has meant critical care provision has drastically changed. The World Federation of Critical Care Nurses (WFCCN) recommends an experienced and qualified critical care nurse should lead every shift, with ventilated patients having immediate access to a qualified critical care nurse [1]. Lessons learned from previous pandemics include recognition that severe staffing shortages adversely impact on nurses' ability to respond to the unprecedented service requirements [2–4]. Across the world, COVID-19 has led to rapid and unplanned expansion of critical care units, with the result that there are insufficient senior critical care staff. In consequence, nurses at all levels are being required to take on new and challenging leadership roles. These range from supervising teams of redeployed staff to managing much larger critical care units. However, the rapidly changing and evolving service needs leave minimal time to train or prepare nurses for unexpected responsibilities and changes in role. It is, therefore, important for all critical care nurses to be aware of leadership issues that may arise during a pandemic and strategies that can be used to maintain safe nursing care.

Leadership in critical care

Just prior to the COVID-19 pandemic, the World Health Organization (WHO) [5] State of Nursing Report identified the urgent need for nurse leadership at all levels. In the challenging and demanding world of critical care, effective nurse leadership is crucial to achieve the best outcomes for patients with complex needs, due to the unique, dynamic and constantly evolving situations that arise in the critical care

COVID-19: A Critical Care Textbook. https://doi.org/10.1016/B978-0-7020-8383-9.00003-8

environment. Traditionally, qualified critical care nurses have developed the ability to provide leadership in core areas. Firstly, the management and coordination of all elements of clinical care for critically ill patients at the bedside. Secondly, as senior and experienced nurses, to lead the safe and effective coordination and prioritization of the critical care unit workload, workforce and resources [6]. Thirdly, senior nurses, may be expected to manage specialist nurses and activities such as critical care outreach, practice development and research nurses.

Shift management includes the ability to assess situations, team functions and capability, setting safe and effective team goals, to identify priorities and lead in decision-making, managing resources to achieve and maintain safe care delivery [6]. To prepare nurses for this diverse and demanding role, a component of all continuous professional development needs to be leadership and management. It has long been recognized that proficient and skilled leadership contributes to team effectiveness and cohesion [7]. During a pandemic, it is crucial that overstretched and exhausted staff, who are working consistently outside their normal roles and responsibilities, have access to effective and supportive leadership. Collins et al. [9] argue that the leadership style used can significantly influence nurses' psychological distress levels [8]. There are numerous definitions and approach to leadership, however, most definitions focus on how the leader provides a vision and energy for their team and works towards clear goals [9]. Effective leadership, as defined by the King's Fund [10], is

The art of motivating people to achieve a common goal. The five characteristics of leadership are: developing and empowering people; fostering a compassionate and inclusive culture; sharing a clear purpose and engaging vision; focusing on impact and outcomes; and encouraging a sense of pride and belonging.

COVID-19 has fractured many of the assumptions and work processes in critical care, with nurses placed in unprecedented levels of high-risk situations which may cause psychological distress [11]. A challenge for leaders has been the scale of the COVID-19 pandemic and the incomplete, continuously changing, and conflicting evidence and guidance [12]. During infectious disease outbreaks the attributes of leaders include being a role model, knowledgeable, flexible, diplomatic, fostering a culture of openness, availability and accessibility, having good communication and listening skills, encouraging, being solution-oriented, and adopting an inclusive and democratic approach [11,13]. However, it is a cause for concern that training has tended to focus on nurses identified for redeployment, while leadership training for critical care staff has been limited.

In a pandemic, transformational leadership assumes a new importance. Transformational leadership was defined over four decades ago by McGregor Burns [14], who argued that this leadership approach focused on meeting the needs and values of followers to motivate high performance to meet organizational goals and lead to success [15]. For transformational leadership to be effective, people need to have a shared sense of purpose, which extends beyond reward-based performance approaches [16]. It is accepted that nurses already have shared visions, morals, needs and values, therefore, in a pandemic there is a shared sense of purpose and commitment to protecting services [17]. Transformational leaders recognize the "individual considerations" by encouraging and supporting followers to achieve [18]. Examples include providing feedback, supporting and encouraging professional development. By recognizing each member of the team as unique and individual, this motivates and encourages the individual to perform. Evidence suggests that, for nurses, it can help to maintain job satisfaction, reduce burnout and facilitate a cohesive work environment [19,20].

Traditionally, leadership training and education have focused on developing effective leaders, with the view that if the leader succeeds then the organization will succeed [21]. However, this approach does not recognize the role of the follower, something Coombes [21] identified as the forgotten part of leadership. Coombes [21] argues that it is important to recognize that although an individual may be identified as a leader, they are also a follower and report to another leader. All individuals must recognize that they are both a leader and a follower and, in a pandemic, roles become interchangeable as the situation evolves. Critical to the success of this approach is for staff to have the confidence, autonomy and ability to raise concerns.

Changing models in critical care nursing

In the UK, best practice guidance currently recommends that accepted and validated pre-pandemic nurse-to-patient ratios should be maintained for as long as possible [22,23]. To respond to the shortfall in workforce demands caused by the pandemic, non-critical care-trained nurses may be redeployed, resulting in critical care nurses supervising a group of redeployed staff and patients. It is recommended there should be a minimum of one trained critical care nurse and one registered health care professional for two level 3 patients, and one trained critical care nurse with one registered health care professional for four level 2 patients (compared to the normal 1:2 ratio) [23].

In this changed model of care, leadership at all levels of the nursing hierarchy becomes blurred, with the nurse in charge providing overall leadership for the critical care unit across extended and different locations, for example, theatre recovery, and wards converted to critical care areas. Critical care nurses (both qualified and experienced) find themselves leading small teams of health-care professionals within a designated area, for example, a bay, and delegating aspects of care as appropriate. These new teams may include senior staff who have chosen to support their colleagues by joining the critical care team and, accepting that it is not their first discipline, they will need to work under supervision. Thus, for the first time, critical care nurses may find themselves supervising doctors, physiotherapists and specialist nurses who would normally be senior to them. It is essential that with these colleagues assumptions are not made regarding critical care competence and that they are fully supported as they embark on their new and unfamiliar role. This also places a responsibility on the nurse in charge to recognize and know how to utilize these staff members while maintaining professional accountability and patient safety.

Non-technical skills

Non-technical skills encompass cognitive, social and personal attributes that compliment professional, technical skills. For a disparate group of professionals to work together, effective teamwork and leadership are crucial. It is essential that healthcare professionals recognize and accept the range of expertise and non-technical skills that the group offers, and how these may influence technical skill performance [24]. In consequence, individuals, regardless of role, need to be aware of the total skill mix across the team and how the non-technical skills in terms of situational awareness impact on decision-making, team dynamics, leadership and task management, and affect the delivery of safe patient care.

Situational awareness

Critical care is a high-stakes environment as patients are complex and many events are occurring simultaneously [25]. Situational awareness is described as the individual's assessment of a situation and how that information is used to plan actions and decisions [24,26]. Therefore, if a nurse dealing with a complex patient or managing a group of patients, each with changing conditions and varying needs, has limited situational awareness this may result in poor prioritization of care and decision-making. To improve situational awareness, which in a pandemic is dynamic and constantly evolving, Endsley and Jones [27] suggest three levels or stages need to be considered:

- Level 1: Perception of elements in the environment using sensory systems to understand what is happening around them.
- Level 2: Comprehension of the current situation to identify what is significant in the situation.
- Level 3: Consider the future courses of action by understanding what is going on in the current situation to identify potential problems that may occur in the future and what actions need to be taken.

Factors which may influence an individual's situation awareness can be categorized as relating to the context, the individual, the task and cognitive limitation and tendencies (Fig. 3.1). Therefore, to improve situation awareness and reduce distractions and errors, the use of checklists and protocols is recommended. Crucial procedures should be described as safety critical and no interruption should be allowed once a procedure starts, for example, during intubation, central venous catheter line insertion, or when double pumping vasopressor infusions [26].

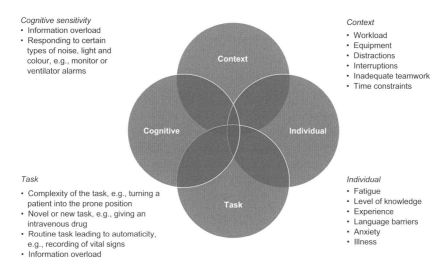

Cognitive sensitivity
- Information overload
- Responding to certain types of noise, light and colour, e.g., monitor or ventilator alarms

Context
- Workload
- Equipment
- Distractions
- Interruptions
- Inadequate teamwork
- Time constraints

Task
- Complexity of the task, e.g., turning a patient into the prone position
- Novel or new task, e.g., giving an intravenous drug
- Routine task leading to automaticity, e.g., recording of vital signs
- Information overload

Individual
- Fatigue
- Level of knowledge
- Experience
- Language barriers
- Anxiety
- Illness

FIGURE 3.1   Factors affecting situational awareness.

Communication

Communication is essential to maintaining effective situational awareness. It has to be noted that prior to the COVID-19 pandemic, an estimated 80% of adverse incidents or near misses in hospitals were due to communication problems [24]. To improve communication among the interdisciplinary team, critical care units may use safety huddles, also termed "take five" or "team huddles". These are short (less than 10 min), stand-up meetings, usually at the start of a shift or at predetermined times to share information [28]. Team huddles follow a predetermined agenda, with the scope of improving patient safety [29]. It has been suggested they are a way to improve staff efficiency and collaboration, and highlight patient needs and safety concerns, and offer staff the opportunity to discuss specific operational issues [30]. During the pandemic, huddles are crucial as they provide a safety net for staff and the opportunity to share and understand the multiprofessional perspectives of patient's needs.

Communication may also be difficult due to background noise, for example, alarms, oxygen hissing, and the wearing of personal protective equipment (PPE). Speaking through a mask can make it difficult for people to clearly hear words. Eye protection may reduce visibly and the field of vision. Non-verbal interaction and cues may be missed and, overall, PPE anonymizes the nurse. Therefore, for patients the wearing of PPE may also add to distress, anxiety and fear; additional challenges include patients with hearing loss and visual impairment [31].To aid communication, gestures, objects, laminated pictures or communication boards can be used. To reduce the anonymity of staff wearing PPE, units may encourage staff to wear laminated photo stickers with the staff member's photograph and name. In addition, different-coloured hats and stripes on gowns may be used to differentiate staff roles and grades [32]. The use of prominent name and coloured role-identification stripes has been reported as being highly effective [32].

Decision-making

This involves critically analyzing and appraising all information within a given situation and delineating a specific course of action or decision [24]. Information needs to be gathered from team members as well as the leader's own personal observation. It is essential that all decisions are communicated to, and understood by, the team; if appropriate a clear rationale should be provided, and team members accorded the opportunities to raise their concerns. Only then can the team work together effectively and safely.

Teamwork

The WHO (2021) [33] defines a team as a

Distinguishable set of two or more people who interact dynamically, interdependently and adaptively towards a common and valued goal/objective/ mission, who have been assigned specific roles or functions to perform and who have a limited lifespan of membership.

As described earlier, the pandemic has resulted in new and different teams forming. It is essential that at the start of each shift the team composition is explored, with strengths and limitations identified. If this does not happen, locum staff and those with limited or no critical care experience may remain anxious and uncertain, which may adversely impact on the care they are able to deliver and the team's situational awareness. Although designed to support patients, the use of photographs and name badges will help personalize the team and through that support integration of members of the team [24].

Task management

Providing care to a group of critically ill patients with a critical care nurse supervising other nurses or healthcare professionals requires effective task management. Critically ill patients require complex care, with numerous tasks needing to be prioritized. The critical care nurse's role is to coordinate, control and manage these tasks. Tasks may be nursing in orientation, for example, intravenous drug administration, providing fundamentals of care, or require input from other professionals, for example, invasive line insertion. Prior to any intervention, appropriate planning and briefing of the team needs to be communicated and checks carried out that all members are clear on their roles and responsibilities during the procedure to follow.

When planning nursing activities, it is important to note that, due to the pandemic, the number of critical care patients will be high, therefore care interventions need to be flexible in order to respond to the unexpected, for example, patient deterioration, an urgent admission or purely the high patient demand. In addition, for critical care nurses, used to one nurse to one patient, prioritizing the workload of a group of patients and other nurses is a skill that needs to be developed. Nurses need to observe their peers carefully for signs of fatigue, stress and distress. Nurses in charge need to take a global view of the overall workload of the unit and recognize the need for their personal support in times of stress and distress.

Professional accountability, delegation, and responsibility during COVID-19

In all clinical settings, during the pandemic, the traditional critical care nurse's role will have changed; however, this does not alter the professional account-ability, delegation and responsibility. It is accepted that the nurse to ventilated patient ratios will be altered, with additional non-critical care staff being rede-ployed to critical care to assist with the care of these critically ill patients [23]. In these circumstances, the nurses professional Code of Conduct must be used to support and guide staff as illustrated below (Fig. 3.2), the elements are inter-linked in provision of safe person-centred care.

Delegation is the process whereby a delegator (e.g., a critical care nurse) allocates a clinical or non-clinical task or duty to another competent individual (delegate). Qualified and experienced critical care nurses will have a crucial role in delegating and supervising other staff. The strength of delegation is that it allows for the most appropriate use of the skills available to provide person-centred care, but it should not be based only on system or organizational drivers [34]. Critical care nurses are accountable for the decisions they make and the tasks they delegate. However, while the delegator retains overall accountability for the management of practice, they can-not be held responsible or accountable for the decisions and actions taken by the delegate. Both the delegator and delegate are professionally accountable for their choices, decisions, actions and outcomes. All healthcare staff (including those not registered) must be aware of, and adhere to, their professional and employment stan-dards and work within organizational policies and procedures [34,35].

The critical care nurse delegating a task or nursing activity must have the authority and competence to delegate the task, and complete an assessment of the need prior to any decision-making. This includes a risk assessment to confirm whether it is appropriate within a given situation and their delegate's competence. They must communicate effectively with the individual to provide clear direction and instruction, confirming their understanding of the task and situation, and checking that they have the competence to undertake the activity. The nurse must then provide supervision, review and evaluate the activity del-egated in the context of the patients' needs, for example; if the patient deterio-rates, it may no longer be appropriate to delegate specialist nursing activities to a non-critical care nurse. The delegate must confirm they accept the activity and communicate the outcome (e.g., document and/or verbally), and understand the

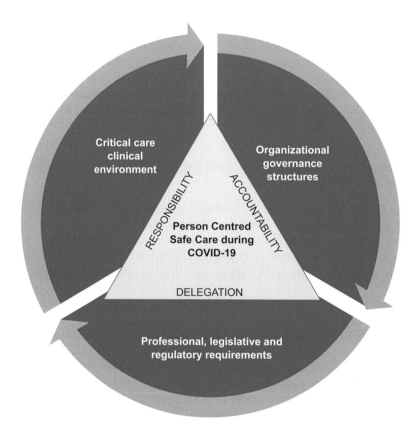

Adapted from: Northern Ireland Practice and Education Council for Nursing and Midwifery, 2020.

FIGURE 3.2   Providing person-centred safe care.

reasons for delegation of an activity. They must immediately communicate any changes or concerns in line with their professional and organizational policies which may compromise patient care [34].

Conclusion

COVID-19 has radically changed how critical care units function. In these uncertain times more than ever, strong and effective critical care leadership is required. Experienced critical care nurses are well able to fulfil this role and are crucial to maintaining the successful running of a critical care unit and patient safety. In pandemics, the uncertainty in peaks and troughs of service need are such that it is impossible to say when critical care units will be able to revert to traditional practice. COVID-19 has led to additional responsibilities requiring senior critical care nurses to lead and supervise a small team of redeployed nurses to care for a group of patients. Experienced nurse leaders will have to adapt and manage larger teams, across an extended critical care unit, as well as continuing with their usual roles and responsibilities. While access to formal leadership training and education is limited, nevertheless, where possible nurses need to reflect on their roles as a leader and team members. This chapter has described some of the leadership and professional issues facing critical care leaders and nurses, providing a starting point for further discussion and reflection.

References

[1] World Federation of Critical Care Nurses. Position statement provision of a critical care nursing workforce. 2019. 22nd March 2019 www.wfccn.org.

[2] Lam KK, Hung SY. Perceptions of emergency nurses during the human swine influenza outbreak: a qualitative study. Int Emerg Nurs 2013;21(4):240–6.

[3] Kang HS, Son YD, Chae SM, Corte C. Working experiences of nurses during the Middle East respiratory syndrome outbreak. Int J Nurs Pract 2018;24(5). e12664.

[4] Corley A, Hammond NE, Fraser JF. The experiences of health care workers employed in an Australian intensive care unit during the H1N1 Influenza pandemic of 2009: a phenomenological study. Int J Nurs Stud 2010;47(5):577–85.

[5] World Health Organization. State of the world's nursing 2020: investing in education, jobs and leadership. 2020. Retrieved from file:///C:/Users/rosse/AppData/Local/Packages/Microsoft. MicrosoftEdge_8wekyb3d8bbwe/TempState/Downloads/9789240003279-eng%20(1).pdf.

[6] Critical Care Networks National Nurse Leads. National competency framework for registered nurses in adult critical care – step 4 competencies. 2018. [UK] www.cc3n.org.

[7] Royal College of Nursing. Leadership. 2021. https://www.rcn.org.uk/clinical-topics/clinical-governance/leadership.

[8] Nielsen MB, Christensen JO, Finne LB, Knardahl S. Are leadership fairness, psychological distress, and role stressors interrelated? a two-wave prospective study of forward and reverse relationships. Front Psychol 2018;9:90. https://doi.org/10.3389/fpsyg.2018.00090.

[9] Collins E, Owen P, Digan J, Dunn F. Applying transformational leadership in nursing practice. Nurs Stand 2020;35(5):59–66.

[10] Fund Kings. Health and care defined. 2020. https://www.kingsfund.org.uk/health-care-explained/jargon-buster.

[11] Crowe S, Fushsia Howard A, Vanderspank-Wright B, Gillis P, McLeod F, Penner C, Haljan G. The effect of Covid-19 pandemic on the mental health of Canadian critical care nurses providing patient care during the early phase pandemic: a mixed method study. Intensive Crit Care Nurs 2021;63:10299. https://doi.org/10.1016/j.iccn.2020.102999.

[12] Rosser E, Westcott L, Ali PA, Bosanquet J, Castro–Sanchez E, Dewing J, McCormack B, Merrell J, Witham G. The need for visible nursing leadership during COVID–19. J Nurs Scholarsh 2020;52:459–61.

[13] Holmgren J, Paillard–Borg S, Saaristo P, von Strauss E. Nurses' experiences of health concerns, teamwork, leadership and knowledge transfer during an Ebola outbreak in West Africa. Nurs Open 2019;6:824–33. https://doi.org/10.1002/nop2.258.

[14] Burns JM. Leadership. N.Y: Harper and Row; 1978.

[15] Collins E, Owen P, Digan J, et al. Applying transformational leadership in nursing practice. Nurs Stand 2019. https://doi.org/10.7748/ns.2019.e11408.

[16] Avolio BJ, Bass BM. Developing potential across a full range of leadership: cases on transactional and transformational leadership. New York NY: Psychology Press; 2002.

[17] Jambawo S. Transformational leadership and ethical leadership: their significance in the mental healthcare system. Br J Nurs 2018;27(17):998–1001. https://doi.org/10.12968/bjon.2018.27.17.998.

[18] Northouse PG. In: Leadership: theory and practice. 6th ed. Thousand Oaks CA: SAGE Publications; 2013.

[19] Balsanelli AP, Cunha ICKO. Nursing leadership in intensive care units and its relationship to the work environment. Rev Lat Am Enfeemagem 2015;23(1):106–13.

[20] Weberg D. Transformational leadership and staff retention. Nurs Adm Q 2010;34(3):246–58.

[21] Coombes M. Followership: the forgotten part of leadership in end-of-life care. Nurs Crit Care 2014;19(6):268–9.

[22] Faculty of Intensive Care Medicine. In: Guidelines for the provision of intensive care services. 2nd ed. 2019. [UK]. www.ficm.ac.

[23] UK Critical Care Nursing Alliance. UKCCNA position statement: critical Care nursing workforce post COVID-19. 2020. https://www.baccn.org/static/uploads/resources/UKCCNA_position_statement_Critical_Care_nursing_workforce_post_COVID_05.05.2020.pdf.

[24] Resuscitation Council (UK). Resuscitation Council (UK). In: Advanced life support manual. 7th ed. 2016. [London].

[25] Lauria MJ, Ghobrial MK, Hicks CM. Force of habit: developing situation awareness in critical care transport. Air Med J 2019;38(1):45–50.

[26] Gluyas H, Harris S-J. Understanding situation awareness and its importance in patient safety. Nurs Stand 2016;30(34):50–8.

[27] Endsley MR, Jones D. In: Designing for situation awareness: an approach to user-centred design. 2nd ed. CRC Press; 2012.

[28] Institute for Health Improvement. Get your priorities straight: tips for using safety huddles. 2019. http://www.ihi.org/communities/blogs/get-your-priorities-straight-tips-for-using-safety-huddles.

[29] Carenzo L, Elli D, Mainetti M, Costantini E, Rendiniello V, Protti A, Sartori F, Cecconi M. A dedicated multidisciplinary safety briefing for the COVID-19 critical care. Intensive Crit Care Nurs 2020;60:102882. https://doi.org/10.1016/j.iccn.2020.102882.

[30] Saint-Louis M. Safety huddles: a safety net for nurses amid the Covid-19 pandemic. Am Nurse 2020. 16 Dec 2020 http://myamericannurse.com/safety-huddles-a-safety-net-for-nurses-amid-the-covid-19-pandemic/.

[31] Nicholls IF, Saada L. Rapid response: communication, Confusion, and COVID-19: the challenges of wearing PPE on a geriatrics ward during the COVID-19 pandemic. Re: Patient Perspective: Gordon Sturmey and Matt Wiltshire. 2020. https://www.bmj.com/content/369/bmj.m1814/rr.

[32] Shurlock J, Rudd J, Jeanes A, Iacovidou A, Creta A, Kanthasamy V, Schilling R, Sullivan E, et al. Communication in the intensive care unit during COVID-19: early experience with the Nightingale Communication Method. Int J Qual Health Care 2020. https://doi.org/10.1093/intqhc/mzaa162. mzaa162.

[33] World Health Organization. Being an effective team player. Patient Safety Education Curriculum; 2021. http://www.who.int/patientsafety/education/curriculum/who_mc_topic-4.pdf.

[34] Northern Ireland Practice and Education Council for Nursing and Midwifery. Deciding to delegate: a decision support framework for nursing and midwifery. 2020. https://nipec.hscni.net/download/projects/current_work/provide_adviceguidanceinformation/delegation_in_nursing_and_midwifery/documents/NIPEC-Delegation-Decision-Framework-Jan-2019.pdf.

[35] International Council of Nurses. The ICN Code of ethics for nurses. Revised 2021. 2021. www.ich.ch.

Chapter 4

Reorganization of critical care services

Chris Carter, Joy Notter

Chapter Outline

In early 2020, the World Health Organization (WHO) declared COVID-19 as a pandemic, with Europe being identified as yet another epicentre (after China, Italy and Iran) [1]. For many countries, this is the worst public health emergency of a generation and has led to the implementation of widespread enforcement measures to help to reduce the spread of the virus. In response, healthcare systems have rapidly adapted services to focus efforts on dealing with the consequences of the COVID-19 pandemic, but it has to be recognized that as current needs continue to rise, existing resources are being stretched well beyond normal usage. As a result, innovative approaches are needed to redress shortages and support the continuance of services. All hospitals have critically ill patients and critical care services, but these were developed to reflect usual service need and not the COVID-19 needs. Evidence from other countries estimates that 5% of patients who develop severe COVID-19 will require intensive care [2]. In consequence, critical care units will be subjected to extraordinary pressure, where patient demand may exceed the available critical care bed capacity.

Critical care before the COVID-19 pandemic

The origins of critical care have been traced to the Crimean War in 1850 when Florence Nightingale separated seriously injured patients and nursed them in

COVID-19: A Critical Care Textbook. https://doi.org/10.1016/B978-0-12-815377-2.00001-9

one area of the hospital, allowing for intensive observation and nursing care to be provided [3]. The practice of grouping the sickest patients nearest to the nurses' station and providing increased observation and intensive nursing care continued for many decades. But it was only during the polio outbreak in Copenhagen in 1952 when hundreds of patients developed respiratory failure that critical care emerged as a speciality. In response to this epidemic, Dr. Bjorn Ibsen, a Copenhagen anaesthetist, successfully treated a 12-year-old girl with severe respiratory failure by inserting a tracheostomy and using positive pressure ventilation. Other polio patients were treated similarly, with medical students providing one-to-one care, resulting in the mortality decreasing from over 80% to approximately 40% [4]. Following the epidemic, Ibsen argued that a dedicated unit within a hospital with one nurse per patient should be developed [4]. This was deemed the start of the modern-day critical care speciality.

Advances in critical care over the past 20 years have led to greater recognition that the care of a critically ill patient often has to start before admission to intensive care, in emergency departments, wards and recovery areas. This has led to ward nurses and doctors becoming increasingly skilled in the recognition, prevention and escalation of care of a critically ill patient. In consequence, critical care units now admit patients who are no longer at the end stage of a disease process, and who will have received time-critical interventions before transferring to critical care. Critical care advances include better understanding of disease processes and evidence to support practices, lung protection mechanical ventilation strategies and better technology including ventilators and monitoring [4].

Intensive care tends to refer to a place within a hospital that provides highly specialized care to critically ill patients, whereas critical care refers to any area where acutely unwell or critically ill patients may be managed, for example, theatre recovery, emergency departments and acute wards. Today, intensive care provision and capacity varies drastically across the globe. In the United States, an estimated 4 million patients are admitted to critical care, compared to England, Wales and Northern Ireland, where an estimated 184,000 patients are admitted annually [5]. The United Kingdom has one of the lowest numbers of critical care beds in Europe [6], with critical care provision classified by levels of care (Table 4.1) [7]. In consequence, critical care services vary between hospitals and may be purely intensive care (level 3) or incorporate coronary care and high-dependency units (level 2), as part of the provision. Intensive care unit (ICU) use either operates an open or closed approach to admission. Open ICUs mean the admitting physician remains responsible for them during the patient's care on ICU, whereas a closed ICU means the patient's care transfers to the intensivist.

Responding to the COVID-19 pandemic

COVID-19 has placed unprecedented pressure on critical care services, which is likely to continue for the near future. There will be ongoing increased staff absence from self-isolation and illness, and the need to refer patients with

TABLE 4.1 Levels of care [7]

Level 0	Care can be met though acute ward-based care.
Level 1	Patients at risk of deterioration or recently relocated from a higher level of care. Additional input, advice and support from critical care may be required.
Level 2	Patients requiring more detailed observation and intervention including single organ support or post-operative care or patients 'stepping down' from level 3 care.
Level 3	Patients requiring advanced respiratory support and/or basic respiratory support with support of at least two organ systems.

suspected or confirmed COVID-19 who develop respiratory failure. This will impact on the availability of extracorporeal membrane oxygenation (ECMO) services where they are available, extending the challenge of preparing and accompanying patients transferring between departments and hospitals for ongoing care. In addition to the relatively high numbers of COVID-19 patients developing severe respiratory failure resulting in acute respiratory distress syndrome (ARDS) and requiring intubation and ventilatory support, the current data suggest an average length of stay for COVID patients in intensive care of 8 days [8].

The role of the critical care nurse and redeployed staff

Critical care nursing is not simply a list of skills or tasks provided to critically ill patients; it requires the nurse to understand the complex needs of each critically ill patient. The World Federation of Critical Care Nurse (WFCCN) [9] defines a critical care nurse as:

'A registered practitioner who enhances the delivery of comprehensive patient centred care, for acutely ill patients who require complex interventions in a highly technical environment, bringing the patient care team a unique combination of knowledge and skills. The role of critical care nurses is essential to the multi-disciplinary team who are needed to provide their expertise when caring for patients and their relatives'.

Using this definition, the nurse is there to provide effective patient-centred care, observing and being proactive in the patient's management, so that any deterioration or changes can be immediately identified and acted upon. This includes being able to cope with unpredictable and unexpected events, explaining all nursing procedures, providing emotional support to patients and their relatives and acting as advocate for the patient. They also play a key role in providing detailed information to other members of the healthcare team, raising concerns, while maintaining and respecting patient dignity and confidentiality [9].

As a result of the COVID-19 pandemic, staff from across the hospital may be redeployed to work in critical care units. To increase the nursing workforce, a pragmatic approach has to be taken, with the first tranche being volunteers, those with previous critical care experience or those with transferrable skills such as anaesthetic and recovery nurses. Staff should be identified early and orientated to critical care before capacity is exceeded and time for orientation becomes impossible. The aim must be to 'best match' the available skill mix to the acuity of patients, with supervision by a critical care nurse, to maintain safe care, even if traditional critical care staffing ratio recommendations cannot be followed for a period [10]. Staff redeployed to critical care should not be expected to work outside their professional scope of practice, independently nursing level 3 patients, unless they are deemed and have been assessed as competent [10].

COVID-19

The critical care nurse needs to recognize that patients who develop severe COVID-19 can rapidly develop type 1 respiratory failure, ARDS and therefore require ventilatory support. In the United Kingdom, an estimated two-thirds of patients who required admission to critical care were intubated and mechanically ventilated within 24 h of admission [15]. In non-COVID-19 patients with increasing respiratory failure the use of high-flow nasal oxygen (HFNO) or non-invasive ventilation (NIV) such as continuous positive airway pressure (CPAP) may be used as a treatment strategy. At the start of the pandemic there was considerable debate over whether HFNO and CPAP were advisable for COVID-19 respiratory failure [16–20]. However, 18 months on, the use of HFNO and CPAP is recommended, but there needs to be close monitoring for clinical deterioration that could result in emergency intubation, which in turn increased the risk of infection to healthcare workers [21].

Where emergency intubation is required, it is a high-risk procedure increasing the risk of transmission to healthcare workers and other patients. Although, increasingly, as a result of the rising demand for intubation, it has to be performed outside of the critical care unit, it is usually carried out by specially formed intubation teams, termed mobile emergency rapid intubation teams (MERITs) [22]. These teams have the requisite expertise to intubate patients in emergency departments and ward areas, then transfer them to the critical care units.

A common feature of severe COVID-19 disease is the development of ARDS: a syndrome characterized by an acute onset of hypoxemic respiratory failure with non-cardiogenic pulmonary oedema resulting in bilateral infiltrates [12]. Internationally recognized ARDS treatment guidelines include conservative fluid strategies for patients without shock following initial resuscitation, empirical early antibiotics for suspected bacterial co-infection until a specific diagnosis is made, lung-protective ventilation, prone positioning and consideration of ECMO (if possible) for refractory hypoxemia [23]. It is essential that fluid strategies must take account of the duration of the illness and the accompanying insensible fluid loss.

Access to specialized services such as ECMO may become increasingly difficult due to the relatively small number of units offering this service and increased pressure on beds. In consequence, the prone position may be used to improve oxygenation. Pan et al.'s [25] cohort study of 12 patients in Wuhan City, China, with COVID-19-related ARDS suggests the prone position may have improved lung recruitability and oxygenation if used early. Anecdotal experiences from centres suggest using the prone position while the patient is on CPAP on the ward, as this may improve oxygenation and prevent the need for intubation. Due to the high numbers of patients requiring prone position, proning teams may be set up to improve efficiency [22]. Traditionally, in ARDS, partial pressure of oxygen (PaO_2)/fraction of inspired oxygen (FiO_2) is used as an indicator of lung function [22]. However, it is suggested in COVID-19, that clinical performance using oxygen saturations, rather that the PaO_2/FiO_2 ratio, should be used [23].

At the time of writing, vaccination programmes are in progress, however, there remains no specific antiviral to prevent or treat COVID-19 and treatment remains focused on supportive care. Several clinical trials are in progress for specific drug treatments, for example, the Randomized Evaluation of COVID-19 Therapy (RECOVERY) Trial [26].

COVID-19 is caused by a virus; therefore, antibiotics should not be used as a means of prevention or treatment. However, it is worth noting that empirical early antibiotics may be appropriate if bacterial co-infection is suspected. De-escalation of antibiotics should be based on microbiology results and clinical judgement [11,22].

Personal protective equipment

COVID-19 is a highly infectious respiratory illness, transmitted through close contact, respiratory droplets and through contact with contaminated surfaces [14]. With high rates of COVID-19 circulating in the community and patients requiring hospitalization, healthcare workers are at repeated risk of contact and droplet transmission during their daily work. Therefore, the use of personal protective equipment (PPE) cannot be overstated, but it may not be 100% effective.

Specialist filtering face piece (FFP) face masks are recommended when dealing with high-risk COVID-19 patients. FFP provides respiratory protection and is worn over the nose and mouth, designed to protect the wearer from inhaling hazardous substances, including airborne particles (aerosols). There are three categories of mask: FFP1, FFP2 and FFP3 (Table 4.2), with the FFP3 respirator providing the highest level of protection and being the only category of respirator legislated for use in UK healthcare settings [13]. Guidance for donning and doffing masks is given in Box 4.1.

TABLE 4.2 FFP protection levels [12]

Filter standard	Filter capacity (removal percentage of all particles ≥0.3 μm)
FFP1	80%
FFP2	94%
N95	95%
FFP3	99%
N100	99.97%

Box 4.1 Guidance on wearing a mask [34]

- Before touching the mask, clean hands with an alcohol-based hand rub or soap and water.
- Take the mask and inspect it for tears or holes.
- Orient which side is the top side (where the metal strip is).
- Ensure the proper side of the mask faces outwards (the coloured side).
- Place the mask to your face. Pinch the metal strip or stiff edge of the mask so it molds to the shape of your nose.
- Pull down the mask's bottom so it covers your mouth and your chin.
- After use, take off the mask; remove the elastic loops from behind the ears while keeping the mask away from your face and clothes to avoid touching potentially contaminated surfaces of the mask.
- Discard the mask in a closed bin immediately after use.
- Perform hand hygiene after touching or discarding the mask – use alcohol-based hand rub or, if visibly soiled, wash your hands with soap and water.

International, national and regional variations in PPE guidance and provision have been identified, providing conflicting information and confusion among healthcare professionals. In addition, potential supply issues with PPE and changes in FFP3 respirators due to the increasing demands, require staff to be fit tested prior to using the new equipment. This may lead to further delays and concerns for staff who have not been trained or measured appropriately for masks and where a sufficient variety of appropriately sized masks is not readily available [27,28]. This concern has already been raised by the WHO [29], who have highlighted that PPE may run out in some countries.

Regardless of the type of PPE worn, one of the greatest risks is prolonged wearing of PPE, as this has been shown to increase fatigue over time, reduce visibility due to the visor and mask and also reduce dexterity due to wearing double or triple gloves [30]. Procedures such as breaking glass ampoules, drawing up medication, performing intravenous cannulation and intubation whilst wearing several layers of gloves and PPE, have been shown to be slower, which in turn impacts on practice [31].

There is also a suggestion that an increased number of healthcare professionals is needed when providing care, particularly in critical care for procedures requiring two nurses to one patient (2:1) when PPE is worn. In addition, staff may need to be rotated to enable them to have time out of PPE and regular breaks, and additional staff may need to act as runners in the clean zone to prepare drugs and equipment and assist with the donning and doffing of PPE [30,31].

The most significant risk of self-viral contamination is potentially during the doffing stage (removal of PPE) if this is done incorrectly. Doffing is a complex, high-risk skill which is often undertaken during periods of stress [32]. During the Ebola outbreak in 2015, studies undertaken during training with a fluorescent marker, showed complex PPE doffing procedures left contamination on hands after PPE removal [33–36]. In consequence, doffing procedures must be clear and simple to follow. Simulation training may provide additional confidence for practitioners to prepare and confirm their skills, as well as increasing expertise in wearing and removing PPE (Figs 4.1–4.5).

Delivery of critical care

To provide an effective critical care service, a specialist workforce, appropriate infrastructure and adequate resources are needed, with critical care units using a multidisciplinary team approach to care. During the height of the COVID-19 pandemic, countries coping with an unprecedented number of patients requiring critical care have to recognize that, as identified in Italy, a major challenge is the risk of collapse in the healthcare system due to difficulty in triaging, allocation and too few critical care beds [13]. Should this occur, the current models of critical care will be unsustainable and a radical adaptation to the delivery of nursing care will be required. Then too, healthcare staff, including physicians and nurses, become infected or exposed, quarantined and unable to work causing additional workforce pressures [13].

Leadership

The reorganization of the critical care services are dependent good leadership. Staff need to be flexible and adaptable, recognizing the changing work practice accompanying COVID-19.

An overall nurse-in-charge will manage the unit, with support from the critical care medical team. Due to increased pressure on hospital services, it may not be possible to maintain an open or closed unit. However, specialist medical input is likely to be required from respiratory, cardiology, surgical and medical teams as appropriate. Strategic leadership will be provided by the matron (also termed head nurse, lead nurse) and the clinical director (lead doctor), who have overall responsibility for critical care services (see Chapter 3 on leadership).

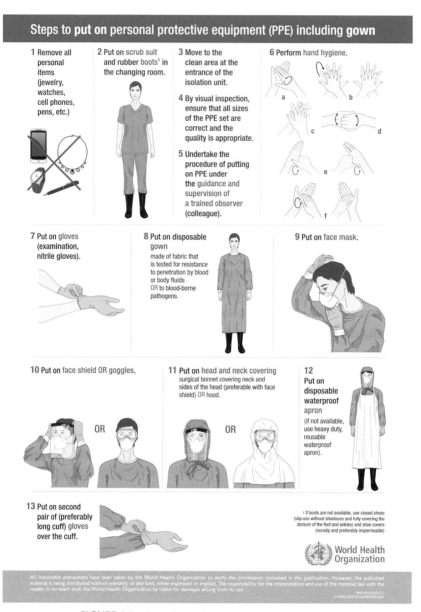

FIGURE 4.1   Steps for putting on PPE when using gowns.

Policies and practice

With the rapid expansion of critical care services, current policies and guidelines may be unrealistic due to the differing levels of staffing, the large influx of new staff not familiar with critical care and the dynamic and rapidly evolving COVID-19 situation. In consequence, maintaining standardized practice and

Steps to **take off** personal protective equipment (PPE) including **gown**

1 Always remove PPE under the guidance and supervision of a trained observer (colleague). Ensure that infectious waste containers are available in the doffing area for safe disposal of PPE. Separate containers should be available for reusable items.

2 Perform hand hygiene on gloved hands.[1]

3 Remove apron leaning forward and taking care to avoid contaminating your hands. When removing disposable apron, tear it off at the neck and roll it down without touching the front area. Then untie the back and roll the apron forward.

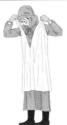

4 Perform hand hygiene on gloved hands.

5 Remove outer pair of gloves and dispose of them safely.
Use the technique shown in Step 17

6 Perform hand hygiene on gloved hands.

7 Remove head and neck covering taking care to avoid contaminating your face by starting from the bottom of the hood in the back and rolling from back to front and from inside to outside, and dispose of it safely.

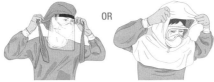

OR

8 Perform hand hygiene on gloved hands.

9 Remove the gown by untying the knot first, then pulling from back to front rolling it from inside to outside and dispose of it safely.

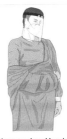

10 Perform hand hygiene on gloved hands.

11 Remove eye protection by pulling the string from behind the head and dispose of it safely.

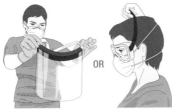

OR

12 Perform hand hygiene on gloved hands.

13 Remove the mask from behind the head by first untying the bottom string above the head and leaving it hanging in front; and then the top string next from behind head and dispose of it safely.

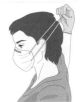

14 Perform hand hygiene on gloved hands.

15 Remove rubber boots without touching them (or overshoes if wearing shoes). If the same boots are to be used outside of the high-risk zone, keep them on but clean and decontaminate appropriately before leaving the doffing area.[2]

16 Perform hand hygiene on gloved hands.

17 Remove gloves carefully with appropriate technique and dispose of them safely.

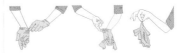

18 Perform hand hygiene.

1 While working in the patient care area, outer gloves should be changed between patients and prior to exiting (change after seeing the last patient)
2 Appropriate decontamination of boots includes stepping into a footbath with 0.5% chlorine solution (and removing dirt with toilet brush if heavily soiled with mud and/or organic materials) and then wiping all sides with 0.5% chlorine solution. At least once a day boots should be disinfected by soaking in a 0.5% chlorine solution for 30 min, then rinsed and dried.

World Health Organization

FIGURE 4.2 Removing PPE when wearing a gown.

supporting staff in practice means guidelines need to be developed, which can include the use of flashcards and care bundles. Flashcards can be used to provide an aide-memoire of key guidelines and core standards relating to care and reflect changes in practice. They may also be displayed to remind all staff of core standards, for example, shift safety checks, guidance for handover, admission process, syringe management and drawing up of infusions.

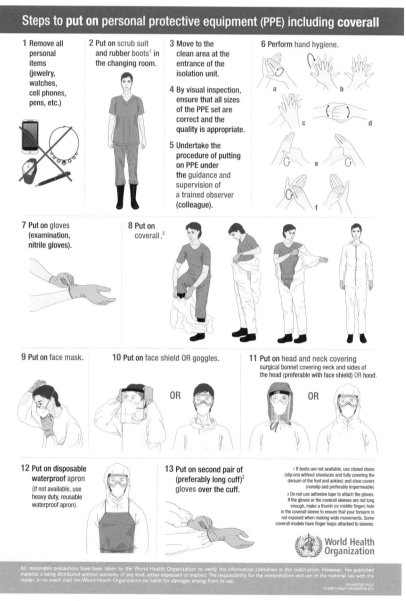

FIGURE 4.3   Steps for putting on PPE when using coveralls.

Care bundles are a series of proven evidence-based interventions relating to a condition or disease that when implemented together can significantly improve outcomes [37]. Each intervention must have a well-established scientific basis and direct the way care is provided. They are presented in practical and easy-to-use formats, which can be followed by all healthcare professionals. Examples

Steps to **take off** personal protective equipment (PPE) including **coverall**

1 Always remove PPE under the guidance and supervision of a trained observer (colleague). Ensure that infectious waste containers are available in the doffing area for safe disposal of PPE. Separate containers should be available for reusable items.

2 Perform hand hygiene on gloved hands.[1]

3 Remove apron leaning forward and taking care to avoid contaminating your hands.

When removing disposable apron, tear it off at the neck and roll it down without touching the front area. Then untie the back and roll the apron forward.

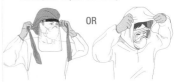

4 Perform hand hygiene on gloved hands.

5 Remove head and neck covering taking care to avoid contaminating your face by starting from the bottom of the hood in the back and rolling from back to front and from inside to outside, and dispose of it safely.

OR

6 Perform hand hygiene on gloved hands.

7 Remove coverall and outer pair of gloves:
Ideally, in front of a mirror, tilt head back to reach zipper, unzip completely without touching any skin or scrubs, and start removing coverall from top to bottom. After freeing shoulders, remove the outer gloves[2] while pulling the arms out of the sleeves. With inner gloves roll the coverall, from the waist down and from the inside of the coverall, down to the top of the boots. Use one boot to pull off coverall from other boot and vice versa, then step away from the coverall and dispose of it safely.

8 Perform hand hygiene on gloved hands.

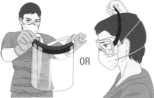

9 Remove eye protection by pulling the string from behind the head and dispose of it safely.

OR

10 Perform hand hygiene on gloved hands.

11 Remove the mask from behind the head by first untying the bottom string above the head and leaving it hanging in front; and then the top string next from behind head and dispose of it safely.

12 Perform hand hygiene on gloved hands.

13 Remove rubber boots without touching them (or overshoes if wearing shoes). If the same boots are to be used outside of the high-risk zone, keep them on but clean and decontaminate appropriately before leaving the doffing area.[3]

14 Perform hand hygiene on gloved hands.

15 Remove gloves carefully with appropriate technique and dispose of them safely.

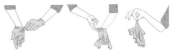

16 Perform hand hygiene.

[1] While working in the patient care area, outer gloves should be changed between patients and prior to exiting (change after seeing the last patient)

[2] This technique requires properly fitted gloves. When outer gloves are too tight or inner gloves are too loose and/or hands are sweaty, the outer gloves may need to be removed separately, after removing the apron.

[3] Appropriate decontamination of boots includes stepping into a footbath with 0.5% chlorine solution (and removing dirt with toilet brush if heavily soiled with mud and/or organic materials) and then wiping all sides with 0.5% chlorine solution. At least once a day boots should be disinfected by soaking in a 0.5% chlorine solution for 30 min, then rinsed and dried.

World Health Organization

FIGURE 4.4 Removing PPE when wearing a coverall.

of commonly used care bundles in critical care relate to ventilator care, central venous catheters and tracheostomy. Care bundles provide consistency in care and can be used as an audit tool to ascertain if they are being followed and the impact on care.

Care planning is an important part of nursing care and follows the nursing process (Fig. 4.6). For COVID-19 patients, the care plan should involve a

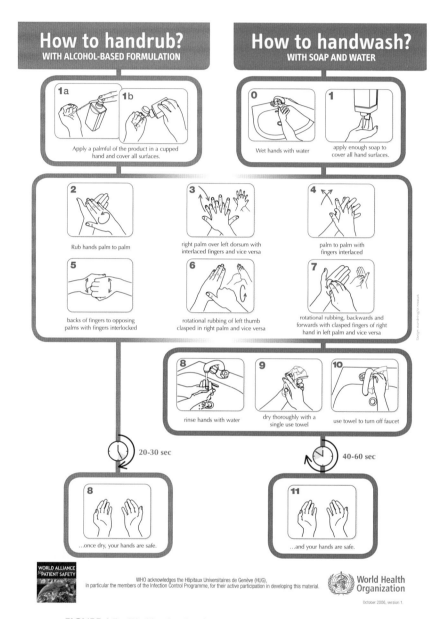

FIGURE 4.5   Washing hands using soap and water and alcohol hand rub.

systematic assessment of the patient and undertaken on admission and at the start of each shift. Goals and the nursing diagnosis are identified, but appropriate plans of care may need rapid revision due to the rate of progression of the disease. Evaluation at the end of the shift needs to review not only if goals have been met, but whether these need changing or adapting, and the best way to

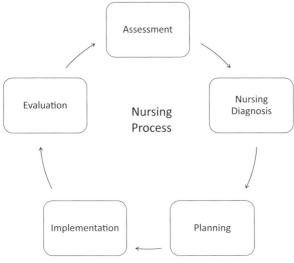

FIGURE 4.6 Nursing process.

utilize the diluted skill mix of healthcare professionals. Due to increased work pressure, such formalized care planning may be difficult, but the critical care nursing process documentation on the 24-h chart must accurately reflect the patient's changing status.

At the start of each shift, a general handover takes place, whereby all patients are handed over, as part of the process nurses are allocated to a specific group (pod) of patients and then a more detailed individual handover is taken. In COVID-19, as a minimum, the bedside handover should include the patient's name, age, past medical history, if the patient has any allergies, reason for admission, length of stay in critical care (number of days), key events that have taken place during the patient's critical care admission, system handover (respiratory, cardiovascular, neurological, renal, liver), next of kin details, a review of the patient's observation chart, drug chart and medical and nursing notes. In addition, a physical check of the patient's name band, infusions and ventilator settings by both the outgoing and oncoming nurse should be conducted to confirm all are correct.

Hospital infrastructures need to be adapted to respond to the increasing demands, which include oxygen, air and power supply and critical care equipment. Oxygen supplies are now under huge pressure, with increased use of ventilators and oxygen therapy being delivered across the hospital. Staff must be made aware of the need to conserve oxygen supplies, reduce hyperoxia and prevent unnecessary waste, for example, switching off an oxygen supply when not in use [24]. Emergency portable oxygen cylinders need to be available. While it is accepted that they are unlikely to be able to sustain a critical failure in walled oxygen supply, they should be readily available to facilitate transfers

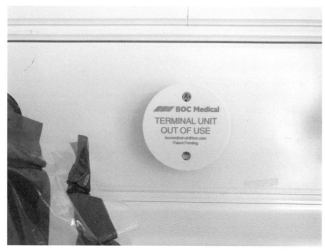

PICTURE 4.1   Walled air supply port closed off to prevent inadvertent connection of oxygen tubing to air flow meters.

and for emergency use. Then too, the increased use of ventilators means there is currently a likelihood of an 'enriched oxygen' atmosphere in clinical areas, increasing the risk of combustion and fire [38]. Fire-preventive checks must be carried out at regular intervals, and any necessary remedial action taken.

In many clinical areas, as a patient safety measure, air supply outlets have been restricted to reduce the risk of connecting oxygen tubing to air flow meters (Picture 4.1) [39]. Most ventilators require piped air supply, with the exception of ventilators used in transport, sufficient outlets and supply will need to be available in locations not traditionally used to provide invasive ventilation.

As the pandemic continues, healthcare services are likely to have to be reconfigured and transformed to respond to the need for a greater focus on COVID-19 to sustain care utilizing staff available for redeployment. However, while this response is seen as crucial, the problem for care providers is that it is essential for healthcare services to be able to respond to non-COVID-19 patients such as those with cerebrovascular accidents (CVA), cardiac emergencies, maternity services, major trauma and cancer care [40]. For hospital managers, the differing needs and approaches to services between COVID-19 and non-COVID-19 critical care availability and input will be an ongoing challenge when planning services and identifying how these patients will be managed.

Summary

Critical care is still a relatively new speciality, which has developed dramatically in the last two decades, and continues to be at the cutting edge of the response to the current pandemic. COVID-19, as a new highly infectious disease with an incompletely described clinical course, results in perhaps the greatest challenge for intensive care since services were first initiated. However, it was developed in response to what was then an unprecedented need. It has become a highly skilled and expert workforce designed to advance care and cope with new and unknown situations. Yet it still retains the ability to transform itself as our understanding of disease processes increases. Treatment strategies will evolve and nursing processes will develop and extend, building on currently used treatments, to meet the unexpected and unprecedented number of patients needing their help, care and support.

References

[1] World Health Organization. WHO Director-General's opening remarks at the media briefing on COVID-19 - 11 March 2020. 2020. https://www.who.int/dg/speeches/detail/who-director-general-s-opening-remarks-at-the-media-briefing-on-covid-19—11-march-2020.

[2] Wu Z, McGoogan JM. Characteristics of and important lessons from the coronavirus disease 2019 (COVID-19) outbreak in China. J Am Med Assoc 2020. https://doi.org/10.1001/jama.2020.2648.

[3] Munro CL. The "Lady with the Lamp" illuminates critical care today. Am J Crit Care 2010;19:315–7.

[4] Kelly FE, Fong K, Hirsch N, Nolan JP. Intensive care medicine is 60 years old: the history and future of the intensive care unit. Clin Med 2014;14(4):376–9.

[5] Intensive Care National Audit & Research Centre. Intensive care national audit & research centre welcomes a new chair. 2018. Press release 4 December 2018 https://www.icnarc.org/Our-Audit/Audits/Cmp/Our-National-Analyses/2018/12/04/Press-Release-4-December-2018-Intensive-Care-National-Audit-Research-Centre-Welcomes-A-New-Chair.

[6] Rhodes A, Ferdinande P, Flaatten H, et al. Intensive care a global problem. Intensive Care Med 2012;38:1647. https://doi.org/10.1007/s00134-012-2627-8.

[7] Faculty of Intensive Care Medicine. In: Guidelines for the provision of intensive care services. 2nd ed. 2019. [UK]. www.ficm.ac.

[8] Zhou F, Yu T, Du R, Fan G, Liu Y, Liu Z, et al. Clinical course and risk factors for mortality of adult inpatients with COVID19 in Wuhan, China: a retrospective cohort study. Lancet 2020. 395. 10229. P1054–1062. DOI.ORG/10/1016/S0140=6736(20)30566-3

[9] World Federation of Critical Care Nursing. Who we are and what we do?. 2019. https://wfccn.org/about-us/.

[10] Platten J. Best practice guidelines for non-critical care staff working in critical care to enable the escalation process only in times of surge. North of England Critical Care Network; 2018.

[11] World Health Organization. Question and answers on COVID-19. 2020. https://www.who.int/news-room/q-a-detail/q-a-coronaviruses.

[12] Sorbetto M, El-Boghdadly K, DiGiacinto I, et al. The Italian corona virus disease 2019 outbreak: recommendations from clinical practice. Anaesthesia 2020. https://doi.org/10.1111/anae.15049.

[13] Public Health England. Guidance: transmission characteristics and principles of infection prevention and control. 2020. 3 April 2020 www.gov.uk.

[14] Li Y, Huang X, Yu IT, Wong TW, Qian H. Role of air distribution in SARS transmission during the largest nosocomial outbreak in Hong Kong. Indoor Air 2005;15:83–95.

[15] Mahase E. Covid-19: most patients require mechanical ventilation in first 24 hours of critical care. BMJ 2020;368:m1201.

[16] Peng PWH, Ho P, Hota SS. Outbreak of a new coronavirus: what anaesthetists should know. Br J Anaesth 2020;395:470–3. https://doi.org/10.1016/S0140-6736(20)30185-9.

[17] Wax RS, Christian MD. Practical recommendations for critical care and anesthesiology teams caring for novel coronavirus (2019-nCoV) patients. Can J Anesth 2020. https://doi.org/10.1007/s12630-02001591-x.

[18] Leung CCH, Joynt GM, Gomersall CD, et al. Comparison of high-flow nasal cannula versus oxygen face mask for environmental bacterial contamination in critically ill pneumonia patients: a randomized controlled crossover trial. J Hosp Infect 2019;101:84–7.

[19] Namendys-Silva SA. In: Respiratory support for patients with COVID-19 infection. vol. 8. 2020. p. E18.

[20] Namendys-Silva SA, Hernández-Garay M, Rivero-Sigarroa E. Non-invasive ventilation for critically ill patients with pandemic H1N1 2009 influenza A virus infection. Crit Care 2010;14:407.

[21] World Health Organization. Clinical management of severe acute respiratory infection (SARI) when COVID-19 disease is suspected. 2020. www.who.int.

[22] Wang K, Zhao W, Li J, et al. The experience of high-flow nasal cannula in hospitalized patients with 2019 novel coronavirus-infected pneumonia in two hospitals of Chongqing, China. Ann Intensive Care 2020. 30. 10. 1. 37. DOI:10.1186/s13613-020-00653-z

[23] Cascello M, Rajnik M, Cuomo A, Dulebohn SC, Di Napoli R. Features, evaluation and treatment coronavirus (COVID-19). StatPearls Publishing; 2020.

[24] NHS England. Clinical guide for the management of critical care patients during the coronavirus pandemic. 2020. 16 March 2020. Version 1.

[25] Pan C, Chen L, Lu C, et al. Lung recruitability in SARS-CoV-2 associated acute respiratory distress syndrome: a single-center, observational study. Am J Respir Crit Care Med 2020. 201.10.1294–1297. DOI:10.1164/rccm.202003-0527LE

[26] Recovery.net. Welcome; 2020. https://www.recoverytrial.net/.

[27] Rankin J. Godzilla in the corridor: the Ontario SARS crisis in historical perspective. Intensive Crit Care Nurs 2006;22:130–7.

[28] Leen T, Williams TA, Campbell L, et al. Early experience with influenza A H1N1/09 in an Australian intensive care unit. Intensive Crit Care Nurs 2010;26(4):207–14.

[29] World Health Organization. Rational use of personal protective equipment for coronavirus disease 2019 (COVID-19). 2020. www.who.int.

[30] Loibner M, Schwantzer G, Brghold A, et al. Limiting factors for wearing personal protective equipment (PPE) in a health care environment evaluated in a randomised study. PLoS One 2019;14(1). e0210775.

[31] Castle N, Bowen J, Spencer N. Does wearing CBRN-PPE adversely affect the ability for clinicians to accurately, safely, and speedily draw up drugs? Clin Toxicol 2010;48(6):522–7.

[32] Casanova LM, Erukunkpor K, Kraft CS, Mumma J, Durso FT, Ferguson AN, Gipson CL, Walsh VL, Zimring C, DuBose J. Assessing viral transfer during doffing of ebola-level. 2018.

[33] Zamora JE, Murdoch J, Simchison B, Day AG. Contamination: a comparison of 2 personal protective systems. CMAJ2006; 175:249–254.

[34] Kwon JH, Burnham C-AD, Reske K. et al. Healthcare worker self-contamination during standard and Ebola virus disease personal protective equipment doffing. In: Open Forum Infect Dis. 3. 1387

[35] Zellmer C, Van Hoof S, Safdar N. Variation in health care worker removal of personal protective equipment. Am J Infect Contr 2015;43:750–1.

[36] Bell T, Smoot J, Patterson J, Smalligan R, Jordan R. Ebola virus disease: the use of fluorescents as markers of contamination for personal protective equipment. IDCases 2015;2:27–30.

[37] Institute for Health Improvement. Evidence based care bundles. 2020. http://www.ihi.org/topics/Bundles/Pages/default.aspx.

[38] Carding R. Hospitals warned of increased fire risk on COVID-19 wards. Health Serv J 25 March 2020. www.hsj.co.uk

[39] NHS Improvement. Supporting information for patient safety alert: reducing the risk of connecting oxygen tubing to air flowmeters. 2016. www.improvement.nhs.uk.

[40] Collins A. London begins major COVID-19 reconfiguration. Health Serv J 18 March 2020. www.hsj.co.uk

Chapter 5

COVID-19 perspectives in low- and low–middle-income countries

Chris Carter, Nguyen Thi Lan Anh, Joy Notter

Chapter Outline

Introduction

In many low- to low–middle-income countries critical care services have evolved and developed relatively recently as advances in medicine have changed and enhanced the possibilities for treatment, increasing the numbers of patients needing intensive care. The nature of the current pandemic has implications for critical care nursing in all countries as, in severe COVID-19 disease, an estimated 5% of patients require invasive ventilation and admission to intensive care, with a further 14% require oxygen therapy [1]. For resource-limited countries this is a major cause for concern, as responding to rapidly increasing patient need in settings with a critical shortage of intensive care beds and specialist staff is extremely difficult. As a result, mortality due to COVID-19 may be higher than the predicted case fatality rate, and it is also debatable for how long low- and middle–income countries would be able to fund the additional critical care costs from their limited budgets [2].

Critical care service delivery

As critical care is a complex, rapidly evolving and developing speciality [3], nurses need to have additional education and training to gain the specialist knowledge, skills and expertise needed. In many high-income countries (HICs) education and training programmes are limited, but in many low- and middle-income countries (LICs/LMICs) the problem is exacerbated by the lack of appropriate courses, and a major shortage of trained and experienced critical care staff. In addition, most training programmes have been developed in HICs with little regard for the very different healthcare systems, settings and facilities their colleagues in LMICs work within [4]. Challenges in utilizing processes from another context are compounded because evidence regarding effectiveness and efficiency of care processes is likely to come from HICs with little recognition that limited access to critical care (for invasive ventilation or non-invasive ventilation) could pose a significant and potentially catastrophic challenge to services. There remains an urgent need for COVID-19-related research, policy and guidelines appropriate for resource-limited settings and differing healthcare systems, with a priority on public health and prevention strategies. As a result, this chapter focuses on some of the issues that need consideration when managing a suspected or confirmed COVID-19 patient in a resource-limited setting.

In many LICs and LMICs, most hospitals are in cities, while the majority of the population live in rural areas, making access to appropriate health care, and assessment of actual need, more difficult. Patients tend to present later in the disease trajectory than in HICs, in part because financial hardship can compound the problem of access to services. Even as countries work to improve access to hospital and critical care, it is becoming evident that their healthcare systems struggle to contain pandemics such as COVID-19, where rapid patient deterioration means that any delay adversely impacts on chances of recovery. In a COVID-19-type outbreak, issues such as enforced local travel restrictions and loss of work add to the problems, with patients struggling to gain access to specialist hospital services, or presenting too late. Unprecedented rises in numbers of patients urgently requiring critical care could overwhelm already overstretched services and staff. In consequence, in planning for future services there may be a need to scale up rural healthcare clinics and hospital outreach services including critical care and expand healthcare service provision in rural areas with high resident populations.

For instance, prior to the peak of cases in India, there were only an estimated 30,000–50,000 ventilators available for the estimated 1 million people, which disease projections had suggested were likely to require ventilation at the peak of a COVID-19 outbreak [5]. This situation fits with other LMICs where evidence also reveals a high burden of critical illness on wards and limited availability of critical care beds. In Zambia, Dart et al.'s [6] audit exploring adult medical and surgical ward patients in a tertiary referral hospital found 45% of patients had objective evidence of need for admission to critical care, yet few had been admitted. From these data, the researchers hypothesized that for the hospital which reported 17,496 annual acute admissions, this equated to 7873 patients requiring critical care input. However, they found there were only eight critical care beds for the whole hospital, findings that were confirmed by the internal audit of Zambia's critical care services which revealed a total of 70 beds across the whole country [7]. These two examples give an indication of the scale of additional resources required to provide comprehensive, sustainable, critical care services. The corollary from this is that inevitably the majority of critically ill patients are nursed on general wards, managed by ward nurses and doctors with limited, or no, critical care training. There is concern that healthcare services would struggle to cope with acute exacerbations and/or patient deterioration when they have little or no way to escalate care provision at short notice [6,8,9]. This affirms the need for context-specific healthcare policy and service provision, with an emphasis on public health and preventing spread of the disease amongst communities.

There is a second and major clinical issue, the very nature of a pandemic means that healthcare professionals have to protect themselves and their colleagues as they strive to care for patients, with what may well be an unfamiliar, and little understood, disease. The current pandemic has shown that few HICs can afford to stockpile personal protective equipment (PPE) and the situation in LMICs is likely to be no better. Indeed, they have the added problem of not having rapid access to increased resources to facilitate acquisition of adequate, appropriate PPE. There is sufficient evidence of the impact of insufficient PPE on healthcare staff, with its inevitable accompaniment of loss of some healthcare workers [10]. This is tragic in any circumstances, but in resource-limited settings, the loss can have additional short- and long-term impacts on healthcare services. Prior to the Ebola outbreak in Sierra Leone in 2014, there were just 70 surgeons and 68 nurse specialists providing care to 5.8 million people through 23 public hospitals [11]. Following the outbreak, the number of healthcare workers reduced, because they either fled, died, or could not work, in some instances because of fear, but in others they were caring for loved ones. While the immediate outbreak was contained and managed, the long-term recovery from this disaster is taking years, hampered by the void left by the loss of experienced healthcare workers [12]. During a pandemic, such as the COVID-19 outbreak, there is a risk that much of the workforce may be unable to come to work due to symptoms, comorbidities, or self-isolation following contact with infected patients. However, it has to be accepted that in societies where there is financial hardship, there is the risk that low-paid staff may need to continue to work when they have been exposed to or have symptoms indicating they are developing the disease.

Nevertheless, resource-limited environments do have a few advantages, and in many such settings, the re-use of the single-use items may be a routine necessity for providing lifesaving care. They are still using strategies that HICs have long abandoned and are now having to reinvent and reintroduce as demand repeatedly exceeds supply. These accepted routine protocols may well need adjusting as with COVID-19 or other such new viral diseases, the length of time the virus can remain live on surfaces and equipment may not be known. Then too, incorrect decontamination or sterilization of equipment may result in iatrogenic spread of the disease [13]. In addition, many of these countries have had experience of managing national and international infectious disease outbreaks, because they regularly face infectious disease outbreaks such as measles, polio and cholera, and as a result are prepared for mass public health messaging, which may prevent the spread of outbreaks and pandemics such as COVID-19, allowing for preparedness and scale-up of healthcare systems. For example, in 2003, Viet Nam was the first country to successfully control the spread of severe acute respiratory syndrome (SARS) [14]. In 2015, the containment of Ebola in West Africa prevented a global spread.

Following their control of SARS, Viet Nam carefully documented the progress of the disease and the policies to manage it and then focused on preparing for any such future pandemics (Box 5.1). They have a significant shortage of healthcare professionals with an estimated eight doctors and 1.446 nurses per 1000 people [15]. As a result, their policies had to be designed to mobilize an integrated, comprehensive response with acute, community and preventative healthcare services acting together as one united workforce. The case study from Viet Nam (Box 5.1) illustrates the importance of government, regional and local preparation, mobilization policies and guidelines that were stringent, but accepted and followed by the whole country. The difference in their outcomes with its lack of fatalities to those of Europe and the United States demonstrates that finance alone is not sufficient to control a pandemic [17]. Viet Nam, because of its past experiences, moved decisively, containing those infected, then testing individuals and contacts early. In recognition of the importance of such rapid action, the WHO Africa Region has been working across the continent to enable countries to scale their readiness for pandemics such as COVID-19.

The examples of success from rapid response to the recent pandemic, even with limited finance, have confirmed the need for countries to be adequately prepared. The challenge of lack of PPE is twofold for countries with limited resources, as firstly, storing PPE is extremely difficult as it means restricting finances for other services. Also, no one could have anticipated the speed at which PPE was used and/or became contaminated. The modern approach of single-use PPE inevitably led to a dearth of equipment, and alternative strategies need to be developed [20]. One practical method that LMICs should adopt is to make their own washable (boilable) scrubs, gowns, masks and hats. There are websites where patterns can be downloaded that are easy to follow for durable clothing that can be used repeatedly. There is also the fact that an unusual element of COVID-19 is the need for total facial protection, with facial visors being expensive. However, it is possible for countries to follow the example of the UK, where volunteers were mobilized to make visors for use in hospitals and communities, and again plans can be downloaded from the Internet. Finally, of equal importance to PPE is hand hygiene, and for countries where running water is not always available, the WHO (2010) [21] has approved a formula for developing alcohol hand gel.

Confirming the diagnosis can also be problematic, given the geographical spread of healthcare services in many LMICs, access to laboratories able to process samples may be limited, therefore in the absence of testing, triage based on clinical case definition or presumptive diagnosis can be used [2]. It is essential that countries work together, sharing information as early as they can to allow for diagnostic indicators of new diseases to be developed and shared. Patients thought to be infected may initially be cohorted in ward areas, although strict isolation must be followed, either using separate rooms or maintaining a minimum 2 m between beds. These approaches are challenging as additional staff will be required to observe side wards and to work on additional wards if they need to

---

Box 5.1 CASE STUDY: COVID-19 outbreak, Hanoi, Viet Nam

In mid-March a large hospital in Hanoi had its first confirmed COVID-19 cases. Three of four inpatient and ancillary departments identified 43 cases of COVID-19. Those testing positive for COVID-19 included healthcare workers, patients, relatives and catering employees, and members of the community following exposure.

The hospital was 'locked down' to localize the epidemic. The hospital had approximately 800 severely ill patients who could not be discharged or referred to lower levels of care. There were over 500 patients with end-stage renal failure who needed dialysis and more than 700 patient family members and 1300 medical staff on duty. The lockdown was for 14 days and implemented by hospital management. Healthcare workers were isolated between shifts in government-designated seclusion accommodation. After 3 days, the hospital was permitted to admit seriously ill patients, and patients needing urgent dialysis were escorted in one by one and then isolated at home. After 14 days retesting was carried out and as no further new cases of COVID-19 were found, staff were allowed to return home and normal services from the hospital resumed.

At the same time, the Ministry of Health (MOH) asked the provincial health services to investigate and review all individuals who had attended the hospital in the 14 days before lockdown. They were given 4 days to do this. In that time all residential areas were tasked with identifying and interviewing all hospital contacts from the identified period. The total number of those screened and managed was 44,293 people. This included 4736 inpatients, 1272 outpatients, 30,515 registered outpatients, 7026 relatives/caregivers, 91 caterers and 653 others. Inevitably, most contacts had come from residential areas within Hanoi (16,714 contacts). Prior to releasing lockdown, approximately 2500 healthcare workers were retested for SARS-CoV-2.

A senior MOH advisor reported the COVID-19 outbreak at Bach Mai had included the greatest number of cases nationwide, but the outbreak had been controlled because:

- Firstly, the hospital was closed to new admissions and locked down, implementing epidemic intervention measures which included isolating all health workers, patients, patients' families, and service providers with deep cleaning of the hospital.
- Second, all healthcare workers, patients, family members and service providers were tested. The results showed that all healthcare workers were negative for SARS-CoV-2, but a number of positive results were obtained, most of these were employees contracted to the hospital.
- Thirdly, the residential localities succeeded in screened everyone who had attended the hospital in the 14 days prior to lockdown. This had been led by the MOH and provincial senior health professionals. Following completion of the investigation and screening, the community localities continued to manage and monitor identified individuals.

Results

COVID-19 is highly contagious, and as healthcare workers, catering staff, patients and relatives move around the hospital they could spread the disease. It was

Continued

Box 5.1 CASE STUDY: COVID-19 outbreak, Hanoi, Viet Nam—cont'd

difficult to identify the first case (F0), but from the total 43 cases, 27 were from the catering company and there was some spread into the community. Those in close contact were placed in isolation for health monitoring, for example, for one patient, this meant her husband, son, mother and maids were all placed in isolation.

In addition, to the 44,293 people tested, a dedicated phone number was released requesting anyone who had not been screened but had attended the hospital to make contact for testing. During lockdown all hospital services were suspended but bodies were still released for funerals. Regulations state that each funeral in an epidemic/pandemic should not have more than 20 mourners.

Conclusion

This case study is a clear example of a successful intervention from a country prepared for unknown and unprecedented infectious outbreaks. It demonstrates the importance of an integrated and coherent policy with guidelines for practice. It affirms the points made previously that it is not finance alone that is essential, but co-operation and knowledge exchange across disciplines and between acute and community sectors. There are lessons for other nations and for planning for future infectious disease outbreaks.

---

be opened. Recognition of the deteriorating patient may be difficult due to lack of knowledge of the disease trajectory, reduced staff on wards and limited availability of equipment. Nursing and medical students may need to be deployed to ward areas and depending on the numbers, to supervise a group of patients and perform vital signs. In these circumstances, it is essential that all observation charts are clear and easy to complete. For example, observations charts may incorporate an early warning scoring (EWS) tool based around core vital signs (heart rate, systolic blood pressure, respiratory rate, temperature and conscious level) [22,23]. Protocols and guidelines need to clearly state that in instances such as severe COVID-19 disease, patients may rapidly deteriorate, and EWS are unlikely to be sensitive enough, as the presenting symptoms mean that these patients will all score highly. In consequence, nurses will need to recognize that every contact counts, they must record vital signs but also look for additional signs and symptoms and record and report any changes in the patient's status.

Observations and any trends they reveal need to be carefully studied to identify patients who require escalation in care [24]. For example, patients who show signs and symptoms of increasing respiratory difficulty should be identified and moved to areas within the wards where increased observation and access to oxygen and emergency suction are available. These areas allow for greater observation and may have additional resources such as oxygen and suction to help maintain oxygenation and reduce further respiratory failure [8].

Access to oxygen is likely to be an issue throughout the hospital system. Ideally, an oxygen plant should supply the hospital, but either this may not be adequate, or it may be absent. Therefore, various oxygen sources including walled, cylinder oxygen and oxygen concentrators may need to be used. In most countries, the onset of a pandemic leads to a reduction in planned and elective surgery and this may facilitate access to additional oxygen sources. However, in many LMICs, hospitals deal with more emergency than elective surgical cases and in these instances access to oxygen is likely to be an increasingly challenging. All healthcare workers need to recognize the importance of conserving oxygen supplies, for example, switching off oxygen sources, when not in use [25].

It has always been recognized that the prone position allows for improved ventilation/perfusion (VQ) matching and reduced hypoxaemia, recruitment of the posterior lung segments due to the reversal of atelectasis and improved secretion clearance [26]. However, pandemics such as COVID-19 make healthcare professionals review their practice, as a result it has been recognized that patients benefit from being placed in the prone position while still conscious. The indications for the conscious prone position include an oxygen requirement of greater than 28% to maintain an SaO_2 92%–96% (88%–92% if risk of hypercapnic respiratory failure) and suspected or confirmed COVID-19 [26]. An added advantage for this is that it requires little equipment and therefore can be utilized for a high percentage of patients while on wards [26].

Nevertheless, all healthcare workers need to check for contraindications such as respiratory distress (tachypnoea respiratory rate >35/min, $PaCO_2$ >6.5) and use of accessory muscles, immediate requirement for intubation, haemodynamic instability, reduced level of consciousness or agitation and unstable spine, thoracic injury or recent abdominal surgery. Relative contraindications that also need consideration include facial injuries, neurological disorders, morbid obesity, second or third trimester of pregnancy and pressure sores/ulcers [26].

The patient should be assisted into the prone position, additional pillows may need to be used to support the chest, a reverse Trendelenburg position may aid comfort, but sedation should not be used to facilitate or maintain proning. Once in the prone position, oxygen saturations should be recorded for 15 min, and vital signs (and EWS) and the patient should reassessed. If the oxygenation improves (SaO_2 92%–96%; 88%–92% if risk of hypercapnia) and there are no signs of distress, the patient should remain in the prone position for 1–2h or as long as can be tolerated. The patient should then be returned to the supine position and nursed upright between 30° and 60°, oxygen should be titrated as indicated. If the patient does not respond to this, the nurse should check that the oxygen is not disconnected or kinked, and/or if using an oxygen cylinder, it is not due to run out. The oxygen should be increased, and the patient's position changed, including side-lying. The position should be discontinued if there is no improvement with the change of position, the patient is unable to tolerate the position and/or there is severe tachypnoea (respiratory rate 35), the patient is looking tired or there is use of accessory muscles [24,26]. In these circumstances the patient should be returned to the supine position and care escalated into critical care.

In all circumstances, including resource-limited settings, the decision to intubate should only be made if a critical care bed is available, with sufficient staffing and equipment. The use of anaesthetic machines may provide a few additional machines. The type of ventilator used will determine the type of ventilation strategy used, but these should include lung protection strategies and all ventilated patients should be monitored. Monitoring will be dependent on the resources available, but as a minimum should include continuous cardiac monitoring and pulse oximetry. The availability of closed suction catheters and viral filters for ventilators may be limited, in consequence, critical care areas are likely to be high-risk areas due to the aerosolization and the requirement to disconnect patients from ventilators to suction [27]. To reduce the risk, every effort should be made to improve air flow, for example, by opening windows if possible.

It is accepted that severe COVID-19 disease may result in the development of acute respiratory distress syndrome (ARDS) [28]. In these situations, it may be appropriate to use the Kigali modified ARDS definition and criteria (Chapter 9). This includes recording any new clinical insult or new or worsening respiratory deterioration within 1 week, SpO_2/FiO_2 <315, no positive end expiratory pressure (PEEP) requirement consistent with American European Consensus Conference Definition. Chest X-ray or ultrasound shows bilateral opacities not fully explained by effusions, lobar/lung collapse or nodules and respiratory failure not fully explained by cardiac failure or fluid overload [28].

As with conscious patients, the prone position should be used in ventilated patients. However, it has to be noted that it needs more staff to reposition the patient and extra resources to manage a patient with severe hypoxaemia. To reduce the risk of aspiration bolus, enteral feeding should be avoided while the patient is in the prone position and gastric aspirates should be measured every 4–6 h.

Complications that may arise as the disease trajectory progresses include renal failure [29]; current evidence suggests that the level of acute kidney failure may be as high as 50% [30], with an estimated 20%–35% requiring renal replacement therapy (RRT) [31]. In hospitals with access to RRT, a system of sharing machines may need to be used. However, this has a cost implication as there is an increased use of consumables and an increased risk of intragenic anaemia due to blood loss from repetitive circuit changes. With limited access to RRT machines other methods of renal support including peritoneal dialysis may need to be used. Acute peritoneal dialysis is indicated in patients who have not had previous major abdominal surgery, stable ventilation and cardiovascular, haemoglobin >70 g/L, activated partial thromboplastin time ratio (APTTR) < 1.3, international normalized ratio (INR) < 1.3 and platelets >60 × 10⁹/L. There are two types of PD catheter, either rigid or flexible [32]. Once the catheter is inserted into the patient's abdomen the peritoneal membrane is used as a filter to remove excess waste and water. Dialysis fluid is then drained into the abdomen and then back out. Contraindications include a body mass index >35, abdominal distention due to constipation and known abdominal aortic aneurysm [30]. The advantages to using PD include lower cost, less consumables required, minimal infrastructure and power, less requirement of highly trained renal staff, releasing them to undertake supervisory and mentoring roles and run continuous RRT machines and it is a lifesaving intervention [32]. Disadvantages include using large volumes may impair diaphragmatic movement and may affect ventilation, particularly if the patient requires non-invasive or invasive ventilation.

As indicated earlier, training of all staff, especially those redeployed, is essential, to respond to the increasing complex needs of patients and demands. Training must include the role of prevention, the need for protection of healthcare workers, together with an understanding of the disease progression, escalation options and palliation [33]. Staff must have preparation and training in controlling symptoms in dying patients, including pain, breathlessness, delirium, agitation and end-of-life care, breaking bad news and access to opioid medicines [34]. It is important to remember the impact these increasing deaths may have on healthcare workers and strategies to support mental health and well-being need to be included in all training programmes. Resources and support could be drawn from staff used to dealing with HIV/AIDS and cancer care. Psychological first aid (PFA) is a tool developed by the WHO to support people after a crisis event. PFA is not professional counselling, psychological debriefing or analyzing what happened. The model involves peers listening to people's stories, being safe, connected to others, calm and hopeful, supportive and regaining a sense of control [35].

In all pandemics and outbreaks, not least COVID-19, lockdowns and international flight restrictions are one of the main challenges for the deployment of experts to support national responses [2,19], although increased access to technology such as Zoom, Skype and Microsoft Teams has enabled countries to share good practice and to develop new initiatives. This is not new, for example, during the Ebola outbreak in West Africa in 2014, identified as a large-scale, gradual-onset natural disaster; initially, the political and international response was slow [35]. In consequence, the lessons learnt have identified that healthcare systems and nurses need to continue to provide care in an already stretched healthcare system, while awaiting additional international help and support. However, it could be argued that recent outbreaks in low- and middle-income countries have meant healthcare systems and personnel are more prepared to respond, but this does not negate the importance of international co-operation and support.

Conclusion

In this chapter, perspectives in the management of severe COVID-19 disease in a resource-limited setting have been explored. In relatively short periods of time, healthcare systems have had to reorganize to prevent the transmission and slow the rate of new infections, for low- and middle-income countries whose healthcare systems are already overstretched this requires a different approach. Care of patients with severe COVID-19 disease must have an evidence base and this must be appropriate for the context in which care will be provided. Therefore, parallel development of evidence-based care from both low- and high-income settings must be developed, with sharing of evidence and lessons learnt.

References

[1] Wu Z, McGoogan JM. Characteristics of and important lessons from the coronavirus disease 2019 (COVID-19) outbreak in China. J Am Med Assoc 2020. https://doi.org/10.1001/jama.2020.2648.

[2] Hopman J, Allegranzi B, Mehtar S. Managing COVID-19 in low- and middle-income countries. JAMA Viewp 2020;323(16):1549–1550.

[3] Endacott R, Jones C, Bloomer MJ, et al. The state of critical care nursing education in Europe: an international survey. Intensive Care Med 2015. https://doi.org/10.1007/s00134-015-4072-y.

[4] Carter C, Mukonka P, Wanless S, et al. Critical care nursing in Zambia: global healthcare integration. Br J Nurs 2018;27(9):497–8.

[5] Centre for Disease Dynamics, Economics and Policy. Modelling the spread and prevention of COVID-19. 2020. https://cddep.org/covid-19/.

[6] Dart PJ, Kinnear J, Bould MD, et al. An evaluation of inpatient morbidity and critical care provision in Zambia. Anaesthesia 2017;72:172–80.

[7] Zambian Ministry of Health. Critical care nursing national needs assessment. Zambia: In Conjunction with Birmingham City University (UK); 2016.

[8] Carter C, Snell D. Nursing the critically ill surgical patient in Zambia. Br J Nurs 2016;25(20):1123–8.

[9] Lillie EMMA, Homes CJ, ODonohue EA, Bowen L, Ngwisha CLT, Ahmed Y, Snell DM, Kinnear JA, Bould MD. Avoidable perioperative mortality at the University Teaching Hospital, Lusaka, Zambia: a retrospective cohort study. Can J Anaesth 2015;62:1259–67.

[10] World Health Organization. Rational use of personal protective equipment for coronavirus disease 2019 (COVID-19). 2020. www.who.int.

[11] Brown C, Arkell P, Rokadiya S. Ebola virus disease: the 'Black Swan' in West Africa. Trop Doct 2015;45(1):2–5.

[12] Holmer H, Lantz A, Kunjumen T, Finlayson S, Hoyler M, Siyam A, Montenegro H, Kelley ET, Campbell J, Cherian MN, Hagander. Global distribution of surgeons, anaesthesiologists, and obstetricians. Lancet Global Health 2015. https://doi.org/10.1016/S2214-109X(14)70349-3.

[13] Iserson KV. In: Improvised medicine: providing care in extreme environments. 2nd ed. McGraw Hill Education; 2016.

[14] Vu HT, Leitmeyer KC, Le DH, Megge JM, Nguyen QH, Uyeki TM, Reynolds MG, Aagesen J, Nicholson KG, Vu QH, Bach HA, Plant AJ. Clinical description of a completed outbreak of SARS in Vietnam. Emerg Infect Dis 2004;10(2):334–8. February–May 2003.

[15] World Bank. Nurses and Midwives per 1000, Vietnam. 2020. https://data.worldbank.org/indicator/SH.MED.NUMW.P3?locations=VN.

[16] Channel News Asia. After aggressive mass testing, Vietnam says it contains COVID-19 outbreak. 30 Apr 20. 2020. www.channelnewsasia.com.

[17] Centre of Disease Control and Prevention. Cases in the UK. 2020. https://www.cdc.gov/coronavirus/2019-ncov/cases-updates/cases-in-us.html.

[18] World Health Organization. African countries move from COVID-19 readiness to response as many confirm cases. 2020. https://www.afro.who.int/health-topics/coronavirus-covid-19.

[19] World Health Organization. COVID-19 situation updates for the WHO African region. 22 April. 2020. External Situation Report 8.

[20] Thomasnet. How to make protective gowns for coronavirus/COVID-19. 2020. https://www.thomasnet.com/articles/other/how-to-make-protective-gowns-for-coronavirus-covid-19/.

[21] World Health Organization. Alcohol-based handrub formulation & production. 2020. www.who.int.

[22] Krysta 1, Kyriacos U, Jelsma J, James M, Jordan S. Monitoring vital signs: development of a modified early warning scoring (MEWS) system for general wards in a developing country. PLoS One 2014;9:e87073. https://doi.org/10.1371/journal.pone.0087073.

[23] Kyriacos U, Jelsma J, James M, Jordan S. Early warning scoring systems versus standard observations charts for wards in South Africa: a cluster randomized controlled trial. Trials 2015;20(16):103. https://doi.org/10.1186/s13063-015-0624-2.

[24] Carter C, Aedy H, Notter J. COVID-19 disease: assessment of a critically ill patient. Clinics in Integrated Care 2020;1:100001.

[25] NHS England. Clinical guide for the management of critical care patients during the coronavirus pandemic. 16 March 2020. Version 1.

[26] Intensive Care Society. Guidance for conscious proning. 2020. [UK] www.ics.ac.

[27] Public Health England. Guidance: transmission characteristics and principles of infection prevention and control. 3 April 2020. www.gov.uk.

[28] Riviello ED, Kiviri W, Twagirumugabe T, Mueller A, Banner-Goodspeed VM, Officer L, Novack V, Mutumwinka M, Talmor DS, Fowler RA. Hospital incidence and outcomes of the Acute Respiratory Distress Syndrome using the Kigali modification of the Berlin Definition. Am J Respir Crit Care Med 2020;193(1):52–9. https://doi.org/10.1164/rccm.201503-0584OC.

[29] EMRIT. Internet Book of critical care. 2020. https://emcrit.org/ibcc/COVID19/#renal_failure.

[30] Bowes E. King's Kidney Care King's College Hospital NHS Foundation Trust Acute Peritoneal Dialysis on Intensive Care Units Protocol 17th April 2020. London. 2020.

[31] Intensive Care Society. COVID-19: a synthesis of clinical experience in UK intensive care settings. London. 2020.

[32] Georgi Abraham G, Varughese S, Mathew M, Vijayan M. A review of acute and chronic peritoneal dialysis in developing countries. Clin Kidney J 2015;8(3):310–7.

[33] Christian R, Ntizimira CR, Nkurikiyimfura JL, Mukeshimana O, Ngizwenayo S, Mukasahaha D, Clancy C. Palliative care in Africa: a global challenge. Ecancermedicalscience 2014;8:493.

[34] Rajagopal MR, Smith R. The arrival of covid-19 in low and middle-income countries should promote training in palliative care. BMJ Opin 2020. www.blogs.bmj.com.

[35] World Health Organization. Psychological first aid. 2020. https://www.who.int/publications-detail/psychological-first-aid.

Chapter 6

Assessment of the critically ill patient

Chris Carter, Helen Aedy, Joy Notter

Chapter Outline

Assessment of severe COVID-19 has to be effective but rapid. Therefore, this chapter suggests an assessment strategy for nurses to use based on the airway, breathing, circulation, disability and exposure (ABCDE) approach. This fits with the expanding complexity of healthcare provision needed in hospitals and increased patient dependency being coupled with limited intensive care and high-dependency beds. Nurses are increasingly being asked to provide complex care to acutely ill adults on general medical and surgical wards and need to develop trans-ferrable assessment skills [1]. Traditionally, many in-hospital cardiac arrests are deemed predictable and preventable, with a progressive deterioration as respira-tory and circulatory failure worsens. With COVID-19, the situation is very differ-ent, with deterioration rapid and, unless treated quickly, difficult to reverse. With COVID-19, patients may present with signs of viral pneumonia [2]. Common symptoms include fever, cough, dyspnoea, myalgia, fatigue and anosmia/dys-geusia (loss of taste and smell). Approximately 90% present with more than one symptom, and 15% present with fever, cough and dyspnoea [3–5].

Although COVID-19 is a respiratory disease and patients often require oxy-gen therapy to correct and prevent hypoxia, patients may subsequently develop systemic complications which must be recognized. Due to the high numbers of patients requiring critical care, many will initially have to be managed in emer-gency departments and acute wards until a critical care bed becomes available.

COVID-19: A Critical Care Textbook. https://doi.org/10.1016/B978-0-7020-8383-9.00006-3

In this chapter, the assessment of a patient with suspected or confirmed severe COVID-19 has been presented initially from a ward perspective, followed by a critical care perspective.

Planning for an assessment

Full personal protective equipment (PPE) as per hospital and national guidance must be worn when assessing a critically ill patient and will depend on the situation, on whether the assessment is for a non-COVID-19, suspected or confirmed COVID-19 patient. Staff should plan ahead as it takes additional time to don PPE, and prepare for potential procedures that might need to be undertaken when working in isolation areas.

All wards should have emergency equipment immediately available, which must be checked daily and restocked following use, as it is crucial for patient stabilization. However, the high number of patients requiring intubation and the high workload may impact on replenishing all stock. Records must be made and senior staff must be informed when insufficient stock is available.

Assessment of the deteriorating ward patient

Regular assessment is essential because of the limited window for rescue. It has to be accepted that the skills of the nurse and the equipment immediately available will determine the depth, detail and accuracy of the assessment. Essential physiological observations for these patients are respiratory rate, oxygen saturations, pulse rate, blood pressure, temperature, conscious level using the alert, confused, voice, pain and unresponsive (AVPU) or Glasgow Coma Scale (GCS), pain score and urine output. COVID-19 has changed the rules, with many patients now presenting with severe respiratory failure followed by a rapid decline in their clinical condition.

In ward settings, early warning scoring (EWS) tools may be used to support regular vital signs being performed. An EWS is a tool to help ward staff to recognize patient deterioration by combining regular observations and calculating a physiological score. EWS can vary between organizations; in the UK, a nationally agreed and validated EWS is used in many hospitals (Table 6.1) [6]. The score impacts on response and treatment, for example, the frequency of observations and necessity for escalation to an appropriate healthcare professional (Table 6.2). Advantages of EWS include its simplicity as only basic monitoring is required; the tools are easy to use and require minimal training, which allows them to be used by all members of the healthcare team regardless of experience. Nevertheless, there are several limitations, including an overreliance on the score, rather than on clinical judgement – a concern with limited appropriate equipment and staff available. It is essential to remember that EWS are only as accurate as the practitioner who records the observations. Also, that calculation of the score does not equate to appropriate clinical action. EWS must only be used by nurses to support clinical judgement and not as a procedure to lead practice [7]. In severe COVID-19 disease, many patients now present with rapid decline, and EWS are likely not to be sensitive enough, as the presenting symptoms mean that these patients will all score highly. In consequence, nurses now need to regularly record vital signs but also seek out additional clinical signs and symptoms, observing trends from the patient's vital signs. The limited availability of critical care beds is such that observations of patients with suspected or confirmed COVID-19 must be designed to maximize treatment possibilities.

TABLE 6.1 UK National Early Warning Scoring Tool.

Physiological parameter	Score						
	3	2	1	0	1	2	3
Respiration rate (per minute)	≤8		9–11	12–20		21–24	≥25
SpO$_2$ Scale 1 (%)	≤91	92–93	94–95	≥96			
SpO$_2$ Scale 2 (%)	≤83	84–85	86–87	88–92 ≥93 on air	93–94 on oxygen	95–96 on oxygen	≥97 on oxygen
Air or oxygen?		Oxygen		Air			
Systolic blood pressure (mmHg)	≤90	91–100	101–110	111–219			≥220
Pulse (per minute)	≤40		41–50	51–90	91–110	111–130	≥131
Consciousness				Alert			CVPU
Temperature (°C)	≤35.0		35.1–36.0	36.1–38.0	38.1–39.0	≥39.1	

Reproduced from: Royal College of Physicians. National Early Warning Score (NEWS) 2: Standardising the assessment of acute-illness severity in the NHS. Updated report of a working party. London: RCP, 2017.

TABLE 6.2 Example escalation protocol.

NEW score	Clinical risk	Response
Aggregate score 0–4	Low	Ward-based response
Red score Score of 3 in any individual parameter	Low–medium	Urgent ward-based response*
Aggregate score 5–6	Medium	Key threshold for urgent response*
Aggregate score 7 or more	High	Urgent or emergency response**

* Response by a clinician or team with competence in the assessment and treatment of acutely ill patients and in recognising when the escalation of care to a critical care team is appropriate.
**The response team must also include staff with critical care skills, including airway management.

Reproduced from: Royal College of Physicians. National Early Warning Score (NEWS) 2: Standardising the assessment of acute-illness severity in the NHS. Updated report of a working party. London: RCP, 2017.

The response may include a specialist team, but the nature and title of these teams varies internationally, for example, Medical Emergency Team (Australia), Critical Care Outreach Team or Patient at Risk Teams (UK) and Rapid Response Team (US). The differences between teams have to be recognized when planning processes and procedures. Critical Care Outreach teams tend to be nurse-led and focussed, with the team responding to a range of patients, which includes follow-up of patients recently discharged from critical care, whereas medical emergency, rapid response teams and patient at-risk teams more often have a medical (physician) lead and focus [8].

Assessment of the critically ill patient

A major change in the assessment process is that COVID-19 patients may be initially assessed by redeployed staff and not a qualified critical care nurse. In consequence, it has to be accepted that under the current regimen, qualified critical care nurses will use assessments made by others, but must themselves assess the patient at regular intervals, not just follow reported changes in status. In the light of this, all handovers must include precise details from the patient's notes, highlighting past medical history, reason for admission, a systematic overview of all physiological systems and any identified key events.

In critical care, at the start of each shift, bedside emergency equipment must be reviewed, and any missing elements replaced so that all equipment is working and accessible. This includes emergency oxygen (oxygen port, water's circuit and/or self-inflating bag) and suction unit with tubing. Patient safety checks include verification of the patient's identification band, confirmation of any allergies, the ventilator is correctly functioning (tubing, alarm limits and settings), and continuous intravenous infusions are running and correct. Also check that all electrical equipment is plugged in and not running on battery. It is best practice at all times, and that includes a shift change, for a nurse to introduce themselves to the patient and explain what they are doing. Even though the patient may be semi-conscious or unconscious due to sedation, they may still be able to hear and verbal communications will help reassure the patient and reduce pain and anxiety [9].

Respiratory assessment (airway and breathing)

In self-ventilating patients, an assessment of airway patency includes whether the patient can talk in full sentences. If they have stridor, audible wheeze or gurgling (noisy breathing) due to secretions in the upper airway, they have the potential signs of a compromised airway. A patient may be transferred to the critical care unit prior to intubation or after being stepped down post recent extubation (the removal of the endotracheal tube [ETT]). It has to be noted that evidence suggests COVID-19 re-intubation rates within 24–48 h are up to 60% higher, therefore delaying initial extubation for longer may prevent re-intubation [10].

Inspection involves assessing the patient's respiratory rate, rhythm and depth. An inability to talk in complete sentences must be recorded, as must use of accessory muscles, tracheal position, any audible respiratory sounds and signs of central or peripheral cyanosis or changes in colour. Tachypnoea, an indicator of illness, in COVID-19 is a crucial warning that patients may suddenly deteriorate [11]. Supplementary oxygen may be required to address hypoxia, with oxygen administration being a simple life-saving intervention. Oxygen delivery methods are classified into two groups, variable and fixed performance. Using variable-performance devices (e.g., nasal cannulae), the amount of oxygen delivered (FiO_2) is unknown, as it is dependent upon the patient's ventilatory pattern. Conversely, fixed performance is independent of the patient's ventilatory pattern. In severe COVID-19 disease, to reduce the risk of aerosol-generating procedures (AGPs), non-rebreath, venturi masks and nasal cannulae are usually used [12]. These have a lower risk of transmission when compared with high-flow nasal oxygen and non-invasive ventilation (NIV) with face masks or hoods and humidified oxygen [13]. The use of NIV and high-frequency nasal oxygen (HFNO) in COVID-19 patients is now accepted as one of the strategies to reduce the incidence of intubation and if used early, may prevent invasive ventilation. Recommended by the World Health Organization (WHO) [14], close monitoring is needed as clinical deterioration could result in the need for emergency intubation and therefore increasing the risk of infection to healthcare workers. In consequence, nurses need to have the competence to care for patients with a variety of artificial airways, recognizing and responding to any complications. Safe airway management of patients, especially those with suspected or confirmed COVID-19 disease, requires careful assessment, planning, preparation, teamwork and formal handover [12].

Invasive ventilation is one of the most common reasons for admission to intensive care, with most patients intubated with an ETT to facilitate invasive ventilation. Care of an ETT includes noting the length of the ETT at the teeth or lips and checking the tube is secure. ETT can be secured using ties or commercially available tube ties, for example, Anchor Fast or Thomas Tube Holders. When using ties, nurses must observe for signs of pressure damage caused, particularly at the corner of the mouth. ETT cuff pressure using a manometer should be recorded every 2–4 h, with the aim of maintaining 25–30 mmHg. This range has been recognized as reducing tracheal damage [15]. There are various modes of ventilation, depending on the manufacturer. It is not the scope of this chapter to discuss each mode of ventilation; however, they can broadly be grouped into three categories. **Controlled or mandatory modes** require the ventilator to deliver all breaths regardless of the patient's efforts, with the ventilator determining the respiratory rate and tidal volume. **Spontaneous modes** allow the ventilator to respond to the patient's effort to breath, but alarm if the patient does not trigger a breath within the apnoea time set. A **combination of the controlled and spontaneous modes** allows the patient to breath spontaneously, but if the patient does not trigger a breath, the ventilator delivers a mandatory breath [16].

Endotracheal or tracheal suctioning removes secretions to maintain a patent airway enabling the nurse to assess the amount, colour and consistency of secretions. Traditionally, respiratory assessment includes verification of the ventilatory parameters, settings and alarms. Patient assessment includes auscultation, respiratory rate, SpO_2, work of breathing, use of accessory muscles, agitation and review of arterial blood gases (ABGs) results [17]. However, auscultation may not be possible due to the challenges with PPE and the risk of cross-contamination [12,18].

Inspection for any signs of pain, chest deformity (scoliosis), swelling, symmetry, tenderness, bruising or wounds is important. Chest symmetry should be assessed by placing the palms of the hand over the thorax and palpating for signs of pain, deformity, swelling, irregularities as the patient breaths in and out. The hand position is then moved to either side of the thorax and around the chest wall [16].

The chest should be percussed by placing a hyper-extended middle finger of a hand onto the chest. Using the middle finger of the other hand strike the middle finger on the chest (the movement should come from the wrist). The finger striking the finger on the chest should not remain in contact as it affects the noise. Listen for hypo-resonance, resonance and hyper-resonance. Positions for percussion in the anterior position include mid-clavicle at the apex, second, third and fourth ribs, and axilla. Positions for percussion in the posterior position include second, third and fourth ribs lateral to the vertebrae and medial to the scapula, continuing to the inferior lateral portion of the lung [16] (Picture 6.1).

Assessing for fremitus is a simple technique used to assess vibration intensity in the lungs by placing the hands on the chest and feeling for fremitus (vibrations) during breathing, which is a sign of partial airway obstruction. In ventilated patients this is commonly due to secretions in the large airway indicating the need for suctioning. It can be used for comparison to auscultation.

Chest radiographs (X-rays) are performed to identify abnormalities that may influence ventilation and diffusion. In COVID-19, chest radiographs should be performed in patients with suspected pneumonia [2], and may show signs of ground-glass patterned areas, as healthy pulmonary tissue is radiolucent (transparent); abnormalities appear dense on the film [19]. In addition, patients who develop ARDS may have bilateral opacities on chest X-rays due to non-cardiogenic pulmonary oedema. Chest X-rays also confirm the position of invasive lines and tubes such as central venous catheters, ETT and naso-gastric (NG) tubes.

ABGs are regularly performed in critical care and are often taken from an arterial line. The indications for ABG sampling include being part of a new admission, ongoing assessment, or if the ventilator settings have been changed. They can also be used if there are signs of respiratory distress (e.g., increased respiratory rate, reduced tidal volumes, reduced saturations or if the patient is clammy and sweaty), acid–base balance, checking of potassium level, pre- or post-procedure, checking blood glucose level and whether the patient is haemodynamically unstable. In COVID-19 patients, these checks are essential as hyperoxia should be avoided [12].

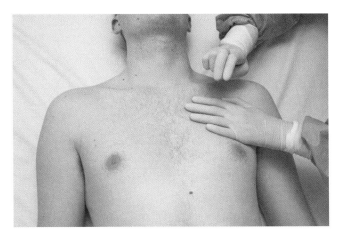

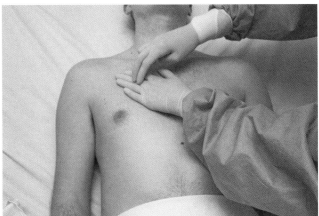

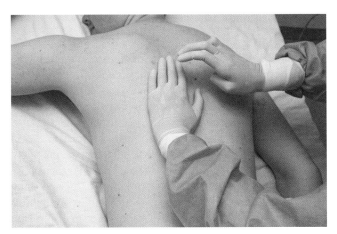

PICTURE 6.1   Percussion of the chest.

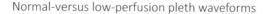

Normal-versus low-perfusion pleth waveforms

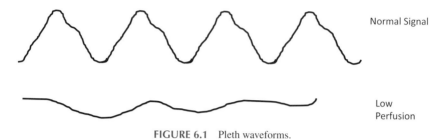

Normal Signal

Low
Perfusion

FIGURE 6.1 Pleth waveforms.

End Tidal Carbon Dioxide (EtCO$_2$) Waveforms

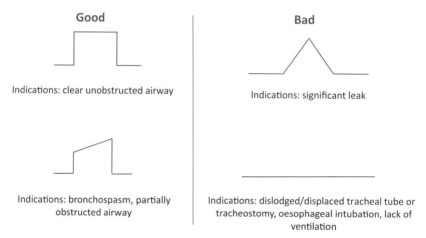

Good

Indications: clear unobstructed airway

Indications: bronchospasm, partially
obstructed airway

Bad

Indications: significant leak

Indications: dislodged/displaced tracheal tube or
tracheostomy, oesophageal intubation, lack of
ventilation

FIGURE 6.2 End tidal carbon dioxide traces.

Pulse oximetry detects a pulsatile signal in an extremity, then calculates the amount of oxygenated haemoglobin and a pulse rate [20]. Pulse oximetry readings do not provide information about respiratory rate, tidal volume, cardiac output or blood pressure, therefore assessment, monitoring and recording of these additional observations is essential [20]. In critically ill patients, pulse oximetry is continuously monitored, it is important to observe the trace to check the waveform (Fig. 6.1). It is worth noting that in self-ventilating patients SpO$_2$ targets of 92%–96% may be used, with lower targets in some patient groups [12].

End tidal carbon dioxide (EtCO$_2$) monitoring detects expired carbon dioxide [20]. It provides an indication of the amount of carbon dioxide in the exhaled air. In a ventilated patient a continuous waveform is monitored to confirm tube position (Fig. 6.2). Normal ETCO$_2$ is 4.5–6 kPa, which is equivalent to pCO$_2$ on an ABG.

Patient positions include supine, semi-recumbent, side-lying, and prone. Most COVID-19 patients will either be nursed proned (to improve oxygenation) or semi-upright, between 30° and 45° as part of the ventilator care bundle to reduce ventilator-associated pneumonia (VAP) [17]. Prone position is commonly used in severe COVID-19 disease to improve oxygenation-ventilation-perfusion, by recruiting increased alveoli in outer dorsal regions of the lung allowing improved distribution of tidal volumes and drainage of secretions [17]. The process involves placing a patient face down and is often performed for patients who are severely hypoxic. Evidence suggests this should be done early and several times if needed [2]. The nurse should note the length of time the patient has been in the position, when the arm position was last changed and any plans for un-proning.

Cardiovascular assessment

Several studies have identified potential distinctive comorbidities among patients with COVID-19 including cerebrovascular disease, diabetes, hypertension and coronary heart disease [21–24]. Fang et al. [14] suggest patients with cardiac disease, hypertension and diabetes on angiotensin converting enzyme (ACE2)-inhibiting drugs should be deemed higher risk for developing severe COVID-19 infection.

Severe COVID-19 disease can cause ARDS, which has a rapid onset and causes severe hypoxaemia, which results in non-cardiogenic pulmonary oedema. Previous medical advice was that fluid balance management should be aimed at there being a euvolaemic (neutral) to a negative fluid balance, particularly in the early phase of infection, in an attempt to reduce oedema [10]. However, often this did not take account of the period of illness prior to admission, which may have included tachypnoea and fever, which can result in a significant deficit in a patient's fluid balance due to insensible losses. Aggressively aiming for euvolaemic fluid balance may cause significant complications including acute kidney injury. In severe COVID-19 disease, renal injury is common and associated with 20%–35% of critically ill patients [10]. In addition, invasive ventilation and the use of high positive end expiratory pressure (PEEP) causes increased intra-thoracic pressure and decreased venous return [17]. This may lead to hypovolaemic shock, clinically presenting with tachycardia, narrowing pulse pressures, hypotension and reduced urine output. In consequence, careful attention to hydration, fluid balance and lower use of PEEP may improve perfusion and prevent complications such as acute kidney injury (AKI).

All patients should be monitored using a continuous electrocardiogram (ECG) and invasive haemodynamic monitoring of blood pressure and central venous pressure (CVP). ECG monitoring provides tracing of the cardiac conduction system. Monitoring in lead II offers the best view and is frequently used as the default setting. A typical adult heart rate is between 60 and 100 beats per minute. A rate of less than 60 beats per minute is termed bradycardia and a rate over 100 beats per minute is tachycardia [25]. In patients who are in the prone position, monitoring is still required; however the traditional lead placement is not possible, and chest leads are reversed, with electrodes placed on the patient's back.

Manual palpation of a patient's pulse should be carried out irrespective of a display shown on a pulse oximetry, automatic blood pressure machine or cardiac monitor. The strength and rhythm of the pulse as well as the rate should be noted, as this may be an indication of stroke volume and peripheral perfusion. Assessment includes measuring the rate and rhythm, also if appropriate assessing peripheral pulse in comparison to the apex beat [16]. If an abnormality is detected, for example, an irregularity, a 12-lead ECG should be performed, and it should be investigated further. Commonly, irregularity of heart rate is secondary to electrolyte disturbances, specifically potassium and magnesium. These bloods should be routinely checked, and electrolytes supplemented as indicated [16].

Blood pressure (BP) is the force or pressure exerted by the blood against the walls of the blood vessels. BP varies throughout the heart and vascular system, being highest in the aorta and gradually reducing with the lowest pressure in the arterioles and capillaries [16]. Pressure is higher in arteries than in veins due to the reduction in pressure as blood is passed through the capillary bed. Ventricular contraction forces blood into the aorta, creating the systolic pressure. This is followed by relaxation as the aorta recoils still maintaining some constriction, referred to as the diastolic pressure. The difference between the systolic and diastolic pressure is known as the pulse pressure. BP can be measured using either a non-invasive (sphygmomanometer and stethoscope) or automated device, or transduced invasively via an arterial line. Mean arterial pressure (MAP) is the average pressure reading within the arterial system. It is generally accepted that a MAP >65–70 mmHg is required to maintain adequate perfusion to key organs, for example the kidneys. In severe COVID-19, patients commonly develop AKI, therefore maintaining an adequate MAP is an important preventative strategy. Automated BP machines record MAP intermittently, in comparison to transduced arterial BP, where MAP is shown continuously.

Non-invasive BP (NIBP) is the most common method of recording blood pressure on wards. This method has limitations, of which nurses need to be aware. These include the accuracy of readings in hyper- or hypotensive states. Potential complications include ulnar nerve injury and problems associated with prolonged or frequent NIBP cycling, such as oedema, petechiae and bruising, friction blisters, failure to cycle and intravenous fluid failure [16]. In haemodynamically unstable patients, the NIBP method is less suitable due to the intermittent measurements given. Invasive BP measurement is the preferred method of assessment in critical care. Arterial BP (ABP) is measured through an arterial catheter inserted into the radial, brachial or femoral artery. When attached to a monitor and transduced, a continuous waveform and real-time BP is provided. ABP is measured by recording the pressure exerted on the sides of the blood vessels, whereas manual BP involves listening for Korotkoff sounds. ABP can be affected by the ABP trace, level of the transducer table, the pressure in the pressure bag and how frequently the transducer has been recalibrated (rezeroed). While the NBP and ABP cannot be compared, they can be a useful tool if the nurse is concerned about the accuracy of the ABP [16].

CVP measures the pressure on the walls of the right atrium of venous return, through the insertion of a central line (also termed the central venous catheter [CVC]) into either the subclavian, internal or external jugular vein. Femoral CVC lines are generally avoided due to the high risk of infection and inability to record CVP. CVP continuously changes, with the average measurement between 3 and 10 cmH$_2$O [16]. During invasive ventilation, the CVP reading may be higher, due to the effects of positive-pressure ventilation. Patients with severe haemodynamic instability and organ dysfunction may require advanced haemodynamic monitoring. Advanced monitoring including Swan Ganz or thermodilution pulmonary artery pressure; echocardiography methods (oesophageal, transthoracic, suprasternal or transtracheal Dopplers); and pulse wave contour methods (LiDCO, pulsion medical system, PiCCO) may be required for patients with severe COVID-19 disease. However, it is not within the scope of this chapter to discuss these methods.

Other aspects of cardiac assessment include measuring central and peripheral capillary refill, skin colour, oedema, temperature, heart sounds and blood results. Capillary refill time (CRT) is a simple bedside test to determine the measurement of perfusion, with normal CRT under 2 s [26,27]. The patient's skin colour should be observed for signs of pallor (pale, cold and clammy), any scars or changes in skin colour, for example, mottled or flushed skin. Signs of anaemia, jaundice and cyanosis should be checked by observing the mucous membranes, for example, inside the lips or lower eyelids [16]. Oedema is caused by abnormal fluid distribution to the third space into the extracellular and extravascular space [16]. To assess oedema, pressure is applied firmly over a bony prominence for 5 s, enabling the severity of the oedema. This is dependent on the depth in millimetres (mm) in the remaining finger imprint and is termed pitting oedema.

A common non-specific feature of COVID-19 is pyrexia (fever), the body's response to the infection [2]. Core temperature should be routinely measured, either via the axilla, mouth or tympanic membrane. Other methods of temperature measurement include rectal, bladder, oesophageal or via a haemodynamic monitor, for example, Swan Ganz catheter or PiCCO. The sublingual route is rarely used in critically ill patients as they are intubated. Any anti-pyretic therapy should be noted as it may mask pyrexia, reducing one of the key warning signs.

Critically ill patients are immobile and at increased risk of developing venous thromboembolism (VTE), which could be reduced with appropriate prophylaxis. In COVID-19 patients, it is unclear if they are at increased risk of developing VTE. Wang et al. [28] found critically ill COVID-19 patients with a high risk of developing VTE had a poorer outcome, and where anticoagulant drugs were used as part of the VTE prophylaxis, they were at risk for bleeding. Assessment of the calves for signs of swelling and inflammation should be undertaken to observe and monitor for signs of VTE. Prophylaxis, including mechanical compression such as VTE stockings, should be prescribed and clotting status regularly assessed.

Routine bloods including renal profile, electrolytes, clotting, full blood count and inflammatory markers should be performed as a minimum daily. Patients with severe COVID-19 may have elevated ferratin, procalcitonin and C-reactive protein inflammatory markers. These bloods should also be taken daily and observed for trends [29]. Elevated inflammatory markers may be associated with secondary bacterial infection and poorer outcome; anecdotal evidence suggests these may be indicators of change [30].

Neurological assessment (disability)

Patients admitted to ICU may have an undetected neurological impairment, due to sedations given, or as a result of conditions such as hepatic failure or meningitis. In consequence, the assessment and monitoring of neurological function is an important requirement for all patients regardless of the reason for admission. Neurological assessment includes the assessment of the patient's GCS and pupil reaction. This should take account of effects from drugs and underlying causes and interventions. In ventilated patients, a 'T' may be used to signify intubation or tracheostomy and recorded in the verbal response box. It is important to note that sedation, analgesia and paralyzing agents are not the same thing. While some analgesics and anxiolytics sedate (and vice versa), the indications for use are different [10]. Patients requiring mechanical ventilation who are heavily sedated and/or paralyzed have been shown to have poorer outcomes that those with lighter sedation [31].

Invasive ventilation without sedation allows for greater interaction, promoting person-centred care [32]. However, lightened or no sedation may cause feelings of vulnerability, anxiousness, fear and loneliness [32]. Finding a balance between appropriate sedation and avoiding over-sedation is complex and differs between patients. Nurse-driven sedation scales, such as the Richmond agitation and sedation score (RASS), allow the nurse to objectively assess a patient's sedation and titrate sedation levels accordingly [33].

Neuromuscular blocking agents may be required to maintain gaseous exchange by reducing extrapulmonary resistance and ventilator dyssynchrony, resulting in improved oxygenation. Paralysis of the diaphragm allows for metabolic rest, reduced oxygen consumption and control of breathing mechanics [17]. Neuromuscular blockage may be required in patients with ARDS as this allows for less PEEP to maintain oxygenation and reduced mortality.

Most patients in critical care will experience pain, commonly caused when undertaking routine critical care, for example, repositioning, endotracheal suctioning, procedures or wound care. Untreated pain leads to impaired mobility, prolonged ventilation, psychological stress and possible delirium. Conscious patients should be encouraged to self-report when assessing pain using validated scoring tools such as the numerical rating score (NRS) 0–10 scale, with 0 being no pain and 10 being the worst pain imaginable. This should be compared with pain at rest and during movement or intervention, including aspects which improve the pain experienced. Ventilated patients may not be able to communicate, and reliance on vital signs to assess pain has been found to be ineffective and a poor judgement on severity of pain. Nurses should, therefore, utilize a validated pain tool such as the Critical Care Pain Observation Tool (CPOT) [33,34].

The risk of delirium increasing mechanically ventilated patients rises each day the patient remains sedated and/or immobilized [35]. Delirium can be triggered by the use of anti-anxiety medications, age, environment (busy, noisy, brightly lit units) and sleep disruption caused by frequently taking vital signs, bloods and repositioning. Risk factors include dementia, history of hypertension, alcoholism or being critically ill at the time of admission [31]. Tools such as the Confusion Assessment Method for ICU (CAM-ICU) are reliable and valid screening tools to assess patients for delirium [31].

Exposure and essential care

With significant pressures on staffing, a potential lack of pressure-relieving equipment and use of the prone position, patients are at increased risk of developing pressure sores. Ideally, patients' pressure areas should be assessed regularly, and a pressure risk assessment tool used to identify patients at risk [36,37]. Prone position is known to increase the risk of complications such as pressure sores, endotracheal tube displacement and loss of venous access [38,39]. In spinal surgery patients, rates of intraoperative pressure sores have been reported as being between 5% and 66% [40]. While prevention of pressure sores may be difficult, every effort should be made to minimize the risk [41].

The fundamentals of patient care, such as assisting with washing, oral care and eye care, are a priority in critical care [42]. However, with reducing nursing-to-patient ratios and the focus on management of organ function, this aspect of care can become side-lined. Every effort must be made to prioritize essential care to reduce the potential for long-term effects and delayed recovery. For example, a complication of sedation and coma is that some patients are unable to maintain effective eyelid closure and are at increased risk of corneal abrasion and oedema [43]. Also, many patients complain of extreme thirst [42,43], therefore oral assessments and regular oral hygiene interventions are essential.

Insertion of an NG tube and early enteral feeding are common practices in critical care, to reduce the metabolic changes that occur due to the stress response, resulting in increased protein catabolism, loss of body mass and higher incidence of complications [44]. However, during the COVID-19 pandemic, hospitals may run out of enteral feeds and have to consider using alternative feeding administration options such as gravity and bolus feeding due to a lack of available pumps. Enteral feeding in the prone position is thought to have considerable risks, but to date there is limited evidence [45]. Best practice guidelines recommend the NG tube should be inserted and position confirmed when the patient is in the supine position. Patients in the prone position, receiving enteral feeds, should be nursed in the reverse Trendelenburg position to prevent micro-aspiration. These feeds should be delivered via a pump, with gravity pumps avoided unless there are no others available. Bolus feeding should be avoided until they are in the supine position. It is important to note that enteral feeding should be stopped a minimum of 1 h before proning/un-proning [45]. Gastric residual volumes (GRVs) should be aspirated every 4–6 h as staffing ratios allow.

It is accepted that the process of assessment can be overwhelming. Adopting a systematic approach to assessment allows nurses to go through a complex step-by-step assessment to prioritize care. Once the assessment has been completed, the information gathered will help to formulate a nursing care plan and tailor each type of assessment in a timely manner to meet patient need. The care plan needs to provide specific, measurable, reliable and timely goals to direct care. At the end of a nurse's shift, care should be evaluated and the result used as a tool for handover and communication during the daily critical care medical rounds.

References

[1] Steen CD, Costello J. Teaching preregistration student nurses to assess acutely ill patients: an evaluation of an acute illness management programme. Nurse Educ Pract 2008;8(5):343–51.

[2] British Medical Journal. Coronavirus diseases 2019 (COVID-19). Best Practice; 2020. www.bestpractice.bmj.com.

[3] Huang C, Wang Y, Li X, et al. Clinical features of patients infected with 2019 novel coronavirus in Wuhan, China. Lancet 2020;395(10223):497–506.

[4] Sun P, Qie S, Liu Z, et al. Clinical characteristics of 50466 hospitalized patients with 2019-nCoV infection. J Med Virol 2020;92(6):612–617.

[5] Chen N, Zhou M, Dong X, et al. Epidemiological and clinical characteristics of 99 cases of 2019 novel coronavirus pneumonia in Wuhan, China: a descriptive study. Lancet February 15, 2020;395(10223):507–13.

[6] Piazza O, Cersosoimo G. Communication as a basic skill in critical care. J Anaesthesiol Clin Pharmacol 2015;31(3):382–3.

[7] Royal College of Physicians. National early warning scoring tool 2. 2019. [London].

[8] Grant S. Limitations of track and trigger systems and the National Early Warning Score. Part 3: cultural and behavioural factors. Br J Nurs 2019;28(4):234–41.

[9] Pattison N. Critical care outreach: capturing nurses' contributions. Nurs Crit Care 2012;17(5):227–30.

[10] NHS England. Clinical guide for the management of critical care patients during the coronavirus pandemic. 2020. 16 March 2020. Version 1.

[11] Intensive Care Society. COVID-19: a synthesis of clinical experience in UK intensive care settings. 2020. [London].

[12] Resuscitation Council, (UK). Resuscitation guidelines. 2020. www.resus.org.

[13] Li Y, Huang X, Yu IT, Wong TW, Qian H. Role of air distribution in SARS transmission during the largest nosocomial outbreak in Hong Kong. Indoor Air 2005;15:83–95.

[14] World Health Organization. Clinical management of severe acute respiratory infection (SARI) when COVID-19 disease is suspected. 2020. www.who.int.

[15] Patel V, Hodges EJ, Mariyaselvam MZA, PeuthererC, Young PJ. Unintentional endotracheal tube cuff deflation during routine checks: a simulation study. Nurs Crit Care 2018;24(2):83–8.

[16] Edwards S, Williams J, editors. A nurse's survival guide to critical care. Elsevier; 2019. Updated.

[17] Barton G, Vanderspank-Wright B, Shea J. Optimizing oxygenation in the mechanically ventilated patient. Crit Care Nurs Clin N Am 2016;28:425–35.

[18] Wax RS, Christian MD. Practical recommendations for critical care and anesthesiology teams caring for novel coronavirus (2019-nCoV) patients. Can J Anesth 2020;67(5):568–576. https://doi.org/10.1007/s12630-02001591-x.

[19] Becker D, Franges EZ, Geiter H, et al. Critical care nursing made incredibly easy. Lippincott Williams and Wilkins; 2004.

[20] World Health Organization. Patient safety: pulse oximetry training manual. 2011. www.who.int.

[21] Yang X, Yu Y, Xu J. Clinical course and outcomes of critically ill patients with SARS-CoV-2 pneumonia in Wuhan, China: a single-centered, retrospective, observational study. Lancet Respir Med 2020;8(5):475–481.

[22] Guan W, Ni Z, Hu Y. Clinical characteristics of coronavirus disease 2019 in China. N Engl J Med 2020;382. https://doi.org/10.1056/NEJMoa20020. (published online Feb 28.).

[23] Zhang JJ, Dong X, Cao YY. Clinical characteristics of 140 patients infected by SARS-CoV-2 in Wuhan, China. Allergy 2020;75. https://doi.org/10.1111/all.14238. 2020; (published online Feb 19.).

[24] Fang L, Karakiulakis G, Roth M. Are patients with hypertension and diabetes mellitus at increased risk for COVID-19 infection? Lancet Respir Med 2020;8(4):e21.

[25] Hatchett R. Cardiac monitoring and the use of a systematic approach in interpreting electrocardiogram rhythms. Nurs Stand 2017;32(11):51–63.

[26] Mayo P. Undertaking an accurate and comprehensive assessment of the acutely ill adult. Nurs Stand 2017;32(8):53–61. https://doi.org/10.7748/ns.2017.e10968.

[27] Ahern J, Philpot P. Assessing acutely ill patients on general wards. Nurs Stand 2002;16(47):47–54.

[28] Wang T, Chen R, Liu C, Liang W, Guan W, Tang R. Attention should be paid to venous thromboembolism prophylaxis in the management of COVID-19. Lancet Haemotol 2020;7(5):e362–e363. https://doi.org/10.1016/S2352-3026(20)30109-5.

[29] Mehta P, McAuley DF, Brown M, et al. COVID-19: consider cytokine storm syndromes and immunosuppression. Lancet 2020;395(10229):1033–4.

[30] Garrett KM. Best practices for managing pain, sedation and delirium in the mechanically ventilated patient. Crit Care Nurse Clin North Am 2016;28:437–50.

[31] Hruska P. Early mobilization of mechanically ventilated patients. Crit Care Nurs Clin North Am 2016;28:413–24.

[32] Tung A, OConnor M. What is the best way to sedate critically ill patients?. In: Evidence-based practice of Critical Care. 2010. Deutschman CS. Neligan PJ. (Editors). Elsevier Inc.

[33] Emsden C, Schafer UB, Denhaerynck K, Grossmann F, Frei JA, Kirsch M. Validating a pain assessment tool in heterogenenous ICU patients: is it possible? Nurs Crit Care 2020;25(1):8–15.

[34] Connor D, English W. Delirium in critical care. Anaesthesia tutorial. World Federation of Societies of Anaesthesiologists; 2011.

[35] Richardson A, Barrow A. Part 1: pressure ulcer assessment – the development of critical care pressure ulcer assessment tool made easy. Nurs Crit Care 2015;20(6):308–14.

[36] Richardson A, Straughan C. Part 2: pressure ulcer assessment: implementation and revision of CALCULATE. Nurs Crit Care 2015;20(6):315–21.

[37] Baldi M, Sehgal IS, Dhooria S, Agarwal R. Prone positioning: remember ABCDEFG. Chest 2017;151(5):1184–5.

[38] Park SY, Kim HJ, Yoo KH, et al. The efficacy and safety of prone positioning in adult patients with acute respiratory distress syndrome a meta-analysis of randomised controlled trials. J Thorac Dis 2015;7(3):356–67.

[39] Grisell M, Place H. Face tissue pressure in prone positioning. Spine 2008;33(26):2938–41.

[40] Kwee MM, Ho YH, Rozen WM. The prone position during surgery and its complications: a systematic review and evidence-based guidelines. Int Surg 2015;100(2):292–303.

[41] Kharameh ZT. Eye care in the intensive care patients: an evidence-based review. BMH Open; 2016.

[42] VonStein M, Buchko BL, Millen C, Lampo D, Bell T, Woods AB. Effect of a scheduled nurse intervention on thirst and dry mouth in intensive care patients. Am J Crit Care 2019;28(1):41–6. https://doi.org/10.4037/ajcc2019400.

[43] Kjeldsen CL, Hansen MS, Jensen K, Holm A, Haahr A, Dreyer P. Patients' experience of thirst while being conscious and mechanically ventilated in the intensive care unit. Nurs Crit Care 2017;23(2):75–81.

[44] Seron-Arbeloa C, Zamora-Elson M, Labarta-Monzon L, Mallor-Bonet T. Enteral nutrition in critical care. J Clin Med Res 2013;5:1. 1–1.

[45] Hardy G, Bharal M, Clemente R, Hammond R, Wandrag L. BDA critical care specialist group COVID-19 best practice guidance: enteral feeding in prone position. 2020. Version 1.0 - 08/04/2020.

Chapter 7

Non-invasive ventilation and high-flow nasal oxygen in COVID-19

Chris Carter, Helen Aedy, Joy Notter

COVID-19 is still described as a new-to-human virus. As a result, its virulence and disease trajectory with mutations now being increasingly detected, and treatment has had to be developed as the pandemic progresses. In all countries, since the disease was first identified, it has been accepted that a high number of patients with severe COVID-19 disease develop acute respiratory distress syndrome and require respiratory support [1]. Defined as type 1 respiratory failure (T1RF), there is hypoxia (PaO_2 <8 kPa), without hypercapnia (carbon dioxide retention or $PaCO_2$) [2], with patients commonly presenting with hypoxia worsening and additional signs such as tachypnoea, increased use of accessory muscles, tachycardia, pale and cold peripheries, sweating, confusion, agitation or reduced level of consciousness and cyanosis.

Early reports from China, during the initial outbreak, suggested that early intubation and invasive ventilation were preferable to delaying care with the use of non-invasive ventilation (NIV) [3]. The problems arising from this were that first, there were limited numbers of ventilators available for the unprecedented numbers of patients and second, weaning patients off ventilation proved to be extremely challenging and not always successful. Searching for ways to address these problems, improved understanding of severe COVID-19 disease has led to changes in the management of patients. Trialled in Italy, as they desperately tried to cope with the pandemic, continuous positive airway pressure (CPAP), a form of NIV, appeared to have a more significant and positive role than initially thought [4]. With improved and enhanced CPAP equipment, it is generally accepted that

COVID-19: A Critical Care Textbook. https://doi.org/10.1016/B978-0-12-815377-2.00001-9

this is of benefit to patients early in the disease process, prevents deterioration and reduces the need for invasive ventilation [4]. NIV assists breathing by supplying a mixture of air and oxygen using positive pressure to help the patient to take deeper breaths, so improving oxygenation without an airway adjunct via a tight mask or a hood. The patient must be conscious, able to initiate their own breathing and maintain their own airway [5,6].

As understanding of the disease has progressed, the use of high-flow nasal oxygen (HFNO) has been increasingly accepted as an appropriate intervention for suspected and confirmed severe cases of COVID-19 disease, although there is still debate on the timing of when to initiate invasive ventilation [3]. It has to be accepted that with high numbers of patients with respiratory failure, the limited availability of intensive care beds and overstretched resources, 'bridging' or holding measures such as NIV or HFNO may need to be used to improve oxygenation prior to intubation [6]. It is also becoming evident that for those remaining conscious, able to see healthcare professionals, and trying to cooperate with them is very reassuring and key to their continuing the ongoing struggle for breath. In addition, the use of the conscious prone positioning has been found to improve pulmonary ventilation and oxygenation (Chapter 9).

There are different types of NIV: HFNO, CPAP and bilevel positive airway pressure (BiPAP). It is generally accepted that NIV is often used in short-term life-threatening respiratory conditions, such as pulmonary oedema or when intubation carries a greater risk than other benefits, for example, patients with chronic T2RF from chronic obstructive pulmonary disease (COPD) [7]. HFNO differs in that it involves the use of nasal cannulae to provide positive pressure to the airways, similar to CPAP. Advantages of using HFNO over other methods include the humidification of oxygen to prevent dehydration of the airway passages and the use of high flow rates to provide carbon dioxide 'washout', resulting in a reduction in the anatomical dead space and oxygen levels close to 100% [8].

Evidence has shown that NIV is not sufficient to manage T1RF in all patients presenting with severe COVID-19 [9–11]. For some patients, while NIV may temporarily improve oxygenation and breathing, it does not change the natural disease progression and is not a replacement for intubation and invasive ventilation [6,12,13]. Nevertheless, there is emerging evidence that there is a place for NIV in the care of patients post extubation. A review of early data suggested that more than 50% of patients have required re-intubation, however, it is now thought that NIV support may bridge support for this group of patients where fatigue remains a significant symptom, and help in breathing is needed to aid recovery [14].

Continuous positive airway pressure

CPAP delivers a constant flow of oxygen at a prescribed pressure, measured in cmH_2O, which remains constant during inspiration and expiration. Intrinsic positive end expiratory pressure (PEEP) is the residual volume preventing

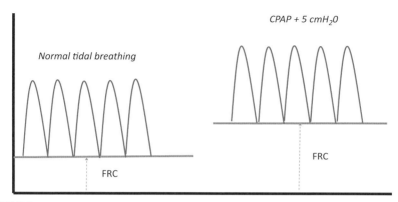

FIGURE 7.1   Increasing functional residual capacity (FRC) with continuous positive airway pressure.

collapse of the alveoli normally measuring around 2.5–3 cmH$_2$O [5]. CPAP is usually commenced at a higher level than normal intrinsic pressure around 5 cmH$_2$O. For most patients with T1RF, it is secondary to conditions that either collapse the alveolar or widen the gap between the alveolar and the blood vessels that surround them, thereby reducing gaseous exchange. The application of PEEP assists in maintaining the patient's airway pressure, prevents alveolar collapse and in turn increases lung volumes and distends them to reduce the distance between the alveolar and the blood vessels to improve gaseous exchange (Fig. 7.1) [5,14,15]. In severe COVID-19, initial CPAP settings have been suggested to be 10 cmH$_2$O and 60% oxygen [15].

For CPAP to be effective, a sealed system is required through application of a tight-fitting mask or hood [5,6]. Both of the methods for establishing a sealed system have benefits and disadvantages. With a face mask, the tight fit means patients may experience pressure damage to the nasal bridge. Newer types of face mask are available with high-volume low-pressure seals that reduce the pressure needed to create the seal when applied correctly, but with rapidly increasing numbers of patients needing CPAP, these may be difficult to acquire. An ill-fitting mask leads to significant leaks, resulting in poor inflation of the lungs, with dry oxygen/air leaking around a mask likely to lead to irritation, abrasions and oedema of the cornea and conjunctiva. The second method, a CPAP hood, requires the patient's head to be fully enclosed with a secure seal around the neck, and the hood can be supported by straps under the armpits [16]. While such hoods reduce the risk of facial pressure sores, when straps are used, they can cause discomfort, pain and, potentially with prolonged use, pressure sores. It also has to be noted that for many patients the noise generated from the high flow required impedes communication with healthcare staff and, for some, causes claustrophobia, which is counterproductive in terms of recovery [5,6]. A potential complication is that gasping breathing and reduced compliance of the lungs can lead to air being swallowed, which if not addressed will lead to gastric distention and vomiting, with a risk of aspiration of gastric contents. In COVID-19-type diseases, patients' lungs are less compliant, and the risk of developing barotrauma and pneumothorax must be recognized. Observations should also be regularly taken and in light of the rapid deterioration that occurs with COVID-19, urgent, early intervention is essential [17]. If positive-pressure ventilation is continued where there is an undrained pneumothorax, it can lead to a tension pneumothorax and potentially cause cardiac arrest [17].

As cited earlier, due to the need for a tight-fitting mask, regular assessment of the patient's pressure areas on the face must be taken, and protective dressings applied if necessary. Note that where there is a nasogastric tube in place, a dressing is more likely to be needed [5]. For both CPAP and BiPAP to be effective the patient is required to wear the mask for extended periods of time to recruit and maintain alveolar distention with the pressure settings. It must also be noted that it is less likely to be effective in patients who have poor tolerance to the pressures and a productive cough as secretions will require frequent removal of the mask for suctioning of oral or nasopharyngeal secretions.

Bilevel positive airway pressure

NIV BiPAP is commonly used in the care of patients with chronic respiratory disease, such as COPD. It may also be useful in COVID-19 for patients who have co-morbidities such as COPD plus COVID-19 (Picture 7.1) [18]. In COVID-19, BiPAP may have a clinical use to improve breathing. However, it carries a risk that inappropriate settings may allow the patient to take an excessively large tidal volume causing barotrauma and volutrauma. BiPAP allows for a high driving pressure coupled with a low driving pressure. This resembles CPAP but provides some additional support. Prior to commencing BiPAP, the patient must be assessed for a pneumothorax, ideally by chest X-ray or ultrasound. Due to the need for personal protective equipment (PPE), chest auscultation for COVID-19 patients is not recommended as it increases the risk of transmission to the healthcare professional [10,19].

Inspiratory positive airway pressure (IPAP) settings can be varied to achieve adequate tidal volumes by allowing patients to breath to a pre-set inspiratory pressure. To achieve adequate tidal volumes, the IPAP can range from 12 to 35 cmH$_2$O (Picture 7.2). Expiratory positive airway pressure (EPAP) works on the same principles as PEEP in CPAP devices, preventing alveolar collapse on expiration, which is maintained above atmospheric pressure. To overcome the difficulty of breathing on a ventilator (including valves) an increase of dead space from the ventilator tubing is achieved by pressure support. Pressure support is calculated from IPAP minus EPAP, and it is recommended that there should be a difference of at least 8 cmH$_2$O [5], with supplementary oxygen provided if needed to achieve oxygenation (Fig. 7.2). Some BiPAP ventilators offer a 'ramp' setting, also termed 'rise time', which allows the pressure to be slowly increased over the first few minutes of ventilation until the required

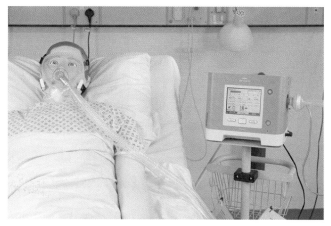

PICTURE 7.1   Bilevel positive airway pressure.

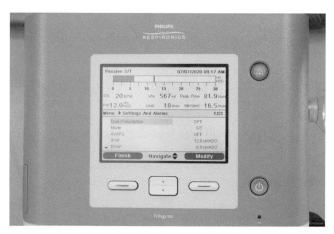

PICTURE 7.2   Bilevel positive airway pressure settings.

pressure is reached. This prevents barotrauma and is considered less distressing for the patient when treatment is commenced. Using this approach, a 25% rise time will take up 25% of the total inspiratory time before the peak pressure is reached [20].

Nursing considerations state that all staff must wear PPE in accordance with national and local guidelines; this includes FFP3 mask and goggles. A well-fitting BiPAP mask should be used to reduce the risk of an aerosol-generating procedure (AGP). Prior to starting treatment, a chest X-ray or CT scan should be reviewed for evidence of bullous emphysema. The patient's weight should be taken or estimated to determine tidal volumes. When commencing BiPAP it may be appropriate to start at low pressures to allow the patient to become accustomed to the machine. IPAP and EPAP can

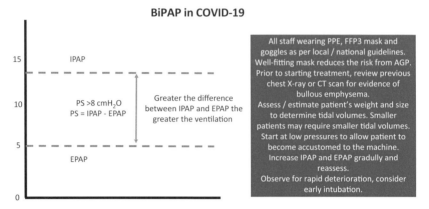

FIGURE 7.2 Bilevel positive airway pressure levels. *BiPAP*, Bilevel positive airway pressure; *EPAP*, expiratory positive airway pressure; *IPAP*, inspiratory positive airway pressure; *PEEP*, positive end expiratory pressure; *PS*, Pressure Support (PS).

gradually be increased and titrated to the patient response. Patients should be continuously observed for rapid deterioration and it may be appropriate to consider early intubation.

Given that BiPAP may be used where there are multiple co-morbidities, decisions regarding escalation in treatment must be agreed prior to the treatment. BiPAP may be used as a trial with a view to intubation if this fails. The treatment escalation plan should have been discussed with the patient and relatives prior to commencing treatment (if it is not life threatening). Patients and families need to be aware when BiPAP is the maximum treatment and should have discussed palliation and end-of-life care [6,7,15].

HFNO

CPAP is the preferred form of non-invasive ventilatory support in the management of the hypoxaemic COVID-19 patient [17]. Slessarev et al. [22] argue that the use of HFNO may meet patient oxygen demands while allowing them to manage their own body positions (Pictures 7.3 and 7.4). This includes self-proning, with chest physiotherapy and intensive nursing care as adjuncts, preventing the need for invasive ventilation. The World Health Organization [3] has supported the use of HFNO in some patients, but recommends close monitoring for clinical deterioration, which could result in emergency intubations, which in turn increases the risk of infection for healthcare workers.

HFNO is sometimes used for patients with increased respiratory effort, for example, tachypnoea, shortness of breath, increased breathing in the presence of hypoxia, evidence of T1RF (PaO$_2$ <10 kPa) and desaturation despite increasing oxygen requirements [8]. However, contraindications include severe respiratory distress, severe cardiovascular instability, unconscious patients, upper airway

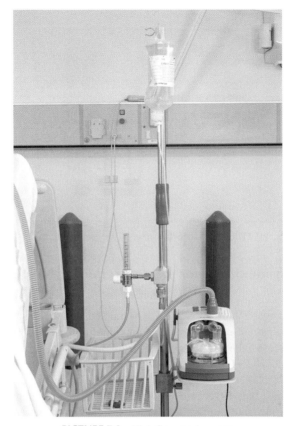

PICTURE 7.3 High-flow nasal oxygen.

obstruction, basal skull fractures, epistaxis and impaired ability to cough or clear secretions. It has to be noted that HFNO dries the lining of the respiratory system. Therefore a humidification water chamber and fluid bag are used and must be checked regularly to maintain water levels and a humidification circuit temperature of 37°C.

HFNO tends to be initially commenced at a flow rate of 60 L/min oxygen to achieve the target saturations (SpO$_2$). Patients must be continuously monitored and vital signs recorded to determine if there is any improvement; the therapy can then be titrated. If there is no initial improvement, oxygen levels should be increased until target saturations are achieved. However, if the oxygen level is >50%, the patient should be urgently reassessed as intubation may be appropriate. It has to be noted that, in COVID-19 cases, the intubation team will require enhanced PPE, which may extend the time before intervention is possible [5,8]. When clinically indicated, oxygen should be weaned first before the flow. When weaning the flow, it should be decreased 5 L at a time or as tolerated by the patient.

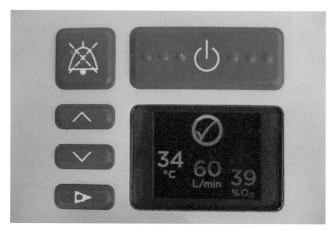

PICTURE 7.4 High-flow nasal oxygen settings screen.

Nursing considerations for patients requiring NIV, HFNO and CPAP

Patients requiring NIV or HFNO must be nursed in specialist settings, with higher nurse-to-patient ratios to support continual observation. As demand for ventilators increases, the ability to procure equipment for use in clinical settings may be difficult [18,24], resulting in staff working with varying types of ventilators and consumables (e.g., ventilator tubing, masks and filters); this raises a patient safety risk. Nurses redeployed or working outside of intensive care units must be given adequate training to care for patients requiring respiratory support using different sets of equipment [25,26]. In addition, as HFNO and CPAP require significant demands of oxygen, hospital oxygen supplies may become depleted, leading to critical failures in availability, not just locally but regionally and nationally [19].

Both NIV and HFNO are classed as AGPs and increase the risk of viral transmission. When disconnecting patients from NIV or HFNO, all equipment should be placed into the standby mode to minimize the spread of the virus in the atmosphere. To reduce the risk of aerosolization, when using HFNO, the patient should wear a surgical mask to reduce particle dispersion, and care must be exercised with viral filters and all secure connections. Healthcare professionals must use enhanced PPE for all procedures, with patients cohorted within a negative-pressure environment where possible [22].

Patient assessment and observations must include continuous pulse oximetry, hourly vital and neurological signs, together with early warning scoring (if used). Added observations include checking for respiratory deterioration, such as increased work of breathing or worsening breathing pattern, use of accessory muscles and mouth breathing, tachypnoea and bradypnoea.

Decreasing saturations and/or increasing oxygen requirements to maintain oxygen saturations must be recorded and reported. Arterial blood gases (ABGs) should be recorded as clinically indicated, but at the least within 1 h of starting treatment and repeated within 4 and 12 h. Patients at risk of further deterioration may benefit from an arterial line that allows for continuous blood pressure monitoring and for ABGs to be taken as clinically indicated [5].

NIV causes raised intrathoracic pressure, which for patients who are haemodynamically unstable may compromise cardiovascular stability through reducing venous return. There may also be challenges with maintaining an appropriate fluid balance, as patients with severe COVID-19 usually present with a history of fever and increased shortness of breath, and they may be intravascularly dehydrated. Insensible losses accrued over the preceding days prior to admission to hospital associated with fever and high respiratory rates will therefore need to be considered and factored in when planning fluid balance. This is crucial because there is a 25% incidence of COVID-19 patients admitted to critical care units developing acute kidney injuries [14].

Periods of NIV should be of short duration to prevent desaturation, but as patients are conscious, they need time-limited breaks to eat and drink, with regular mouth care to prevent problems from dry and sore mouths. Nutritional supplements may be required if there is poor oral dietary intake, and nasogastric (NG) feeding may need to be considered. However, as conscious proning is being increasingly used, NG feeds need to be stopped prior to position changes and gastric aspirates monitored. In addition, care must be taken to avoid patients lying supine with continuous enteral feeds running, as this increases the risk of pulmonary aspiration [27].

Conclusion

As the pandemic has evolved the use of CPAP and HFNO has become increasingly accepted as an appropriate treatment for some patients. In any pandemic where there is incomplete knowledge of the disease trajectory and patient complications, all available respiratory support options have to be considered and trialled. For instance, CPAP was only considered in Italy to address the limited number of ventilators but has been shown to play a positive role for some patients. It cannot and does not replace invasive ventilation, but it may, if used early, reduce deterioration to the point that invasive ventilation is not required.

References

[1] Vardhana SA, Wolchokk JD. The many faces of the anti-COVID immune response. J Exp Med 2020;217(6):1–10.
[2] Dougherty L, Lister S, West-Oram A. In: Royal Marsden Hospital Manual of Clinical Procedures. Blackwell Science; 2015.

[3] World Health Organization. Clinical management of severe acute respiratory infection (SARI) when COVID-19 disease is suspected. 2020. www.who.int.

[4] Intensive Care Society. Use of continuous positive airway pressure (CPAP) for COVID-19 positive patients. 2020. [UK] www.ics.ac.

[5] Edwards S, Williams J. In: A nurse's survival guide to critical care. Elsevier; 2019. Updated.

[6] Davies M, Allen M, Bentley A, Bourke SC, Creagh-Brown B, D'Oliveiro R, Glossop A, Gray A, Jacobs P, Mahadeva R, Moses R, Setchfield I. British Thoracic Society Quality Standards for acute non-invasive ventilation in adults. BMJ Open Resp Res 2018;5. e000283. https://doi.org/10.1136/bmjresp-2018-000283.

[7] Davidson AC, Banham S, Elliott M, et al. BTS/ICS guideline for the ventilatory management of acute hypercapnic respiratory failure in adults. Thorax 2016;71:ii1–35.

[8] Ashraf-Kashani N, Kumar R. High-flow nasal oxygen therapy. BJA Educ 2017;17(2):63–7.

[9] Peng PWH, Ho P, Hota SS. Outbreak of a new coronavirus: what anaesthetists should know. Br J Anaesth 2020;395:470–3. https://doi.org/10.1016/S0140-6736(20)30185-9.

[10] Wax RS, Christian MD. Practical recommendations for critical care and anesthesiology teams caring for novel coronavirus (2019-nCoV) patients. Can J Anesth 2020. https://doi.org/10.1007/s12630-02001591-x.

[11] Leung CCH, Joynt GM, Gomersall CD, et al. Comparison of high-flow nasal cannula versus oxygen face mask for environmental bacterial contamination in critically ill pneumonia patients: a randomized controlled crossover trial. J Hosp Infect 2019;101:84–7.

[12] Namendys-Silva SA. Respiratory support for patients with COVID-19 infection, vol. 8. 2020. p. E18.

[13] Namendys-Silva SA, Hernández-Garay M, Rivero-Sigarroa E. Non-invasive ventilation for critically ill patients with pandemic H1N1 2009 influenza A virus infection. Crit Care 2010;14:407.

[14] Intensive Care Society. COVID-19: a synthesis of clinical experience in UK intensive care settings. 2020. [London].

[15] NHS England. Specialty guides for patient management during the coronavirus pandemic: guidance for the role and use of non-invasive respiratory support in adult patients with COVID19 (confirmed or suspected) 6 April 2020. 2020. Version 3.

[16] Brambilla AM, Aliberti S, Prina E, Nicoli F, Del Forno M, Nava S, Ferrari G, Corradi F, Pelosi P, Bignamini A, Tarsia P, Cosentini R. Helmet CPAP vs. oxygen therapy in severe hypoxemic respiratory failure due to pneumonia. Intensive Care Med 2014;40(7):942–9. https://doi.org/10.1007/s00134-014-3325-5.

[17] NHS England. Guidance for the role and use of non-invasive respiratory support in adult patients with COVID19 (confirmed or suspected) 6 April 2020. 2020. Version 3 www.england. nhs. [UK].

[18] Whittle JS, Pavlov I, Sacchetti AD, Atwood C, Rosenberg MS. Respiratory support for adult patients with COVID-19. JACEP Open 2020;1:95–101.

[19] NHS England. Clinical guide for the management of critical care patients during the coronavirus pandemic. 2020. 16 March 2020. Version 1.

[20] For doctors, by doctors. Learn more about NIV and CPAP. 2020. http://www.fordoctorsbydoctors.co.uk/home/practical-nivcpap-training-day/learn-more-about-niv-cpap.

[21] Lyons C, Callaghan M. The use of high-flow nasal oxygen in COVID-19. Anaesthesia 2020. https://doi.org/10.1111/anae.15073. Editorial.

[22] Slessarev M, Ondrejicka M, Arntfield R. Patient self-proning with high-flow nasal cannula improves oxygenation in COVID-19 pneumonia. Can J Anaesth 2020. 67. 1288–1290.

[23] Wang K, Zhao W, Li J, et al. The experience of high-flow nasal cannula in hospitalized patients with 2019 novel coronavirus-infected pneumonia in two hospitals of Chongqing, China. Ann Intensive Care 2020;30(10):1–37.

[24] Philips. COVID-19: how to safely optimise NIV therapy. 2020. https://www.philips.com/a-w/about/news/archive/blogs/innovation-matters/2020/20200325-covid-19-how-to-safely-optimize-niv-therapy.html.

[25] UK Critical Care Nurse Alliance. UKCCNA position statement: critical care nursing workforce post COVID-19. 2020. https://www.baccn.org/static/uploads/resources/UKCCNA_position_statement_Critical_Care_nursing_workforce_post_COVID_05.05.2020.pdf.

[26] Royal College of Nursing. Guidance on redeployment – COVID-19. 2020. https://www.rcn.org.uk/clinical-topics/infection-prevention-and-control/novel-coronavirus/rcn-guidance-on-redeployment-covid-19.

[27] Hardy G, Bharal M, Clemente R, Hammond R, Wandrag L. BDA critical care specialist group COVID-19 best practice guidance: enteral feeding in prone position. 2020. Version 1.0 - 08/04/2020.

Chapter 8

Invasive ventilation in COVID-19

Chris Carter, Michelle Osborn, Gifty Agagah, Helen Aedy, Joy Notter

Chapter Outline

Hypoxia and the need for invasive ventilation are frequently the main reasons for critically ill patients requiring transfer to the critical care unit. Competence in this area is crucial, with research into the nurse's role in the management of patients on invasive ventilation showing that high-quality nursing care can positively affect outcomes and prevent complications [1–3]. However, invasive ventilation has been identified as an area of practice where nurses feel least competent [4]. Therefore, in this chapter, topics including optimizing oxygenation and prevention of complications of invasive ventilation in relation to severe COVID-19 infection have been fully explored.

Where respiratory failure requires emergency tracheal intubation (passing of an endotracheal tube [ETT] into the trachea) for patients with COVID-19, it is a high-risk procedure, increasing viral load to healthcare workers and other patients. Prior to COVID-19, intubation was normally performed in controlled environments such as the anaesthetic room, resuscitation room and critical care units [5]. Due to the rapid increase in the numbers of patients, and the acute deterioration associated with severe COVID-19 infection, it is now frequently performed outside of the critical care unit by specially formed intubation teams [6]. It must be noted that this is a high-risk procedure for complications such as oesophageal intubation or difficult airway ('can't intubate, can't ventilate') [5].

COVID-19: A Critical Care Textbook. https://doi.org/10.1016/B978-0-7020-8383-9.00008-7

99

In consequence, staff in emergency departments and ward areas may now be required to manage deteriorating patients that require advanced airway management, until the intubation team is assembled or available. As COVID-19 patients deteriorate rapidly, they may be judged as being at increased risk of gastric aspiration and for this group, rapid sequence induction (RSI) is used. RSI also has the advantage that it can minimize the apnoea time during which significant aerosolization through use of facemask ventilation occurs.

During RSI, there should be minimal staff in the vicinity to reduce risks from exposure, with the team including the intubator, an assistant and someone to administer the drugs. In case of an emergency, a runner outside the room should also be available. In addition, all staff need to be wearing appropriate personal protective equipment (PPE) for an aerosol-generating procedure (AGP) [7]. The procedure involves inducing loss of consciousness (by use of drugs), application of cricoid pressure, insertion of an ETT and confirmation of tube position. ETTs come in varying sizes and are either cuffed or uncuffed. Adult tubes are cuffed, whereas uncuffed tubes are used in children under 8 years old to prevent excessive pressure on tracheal tissue.

Regarding the decision to intubate a suspected or confirmed COVID-19 patient, there are procedural and medical issues to be taken into consideration. Any airway intervention should be managed electively rather than as an emergency [8]. In consequence, protocols, and cognitive aids such as checklists, cross-checking and preplanning for all eventualities including difficult airway scenarios should be discussed and agreed prior to the procedure [8]. Prior to intubation, the patient should be preoxygenated with 100% oxygen using a bag, valve mask (ambu bag) or anaesthetic circuit. A two-person technique should be used, to achieve a better seal, and to reduce the risk of aerosolization.

Potential complications include right main bronchus intubation, lacerated lips, tongue, pharynx and trachea, vocal cord injury, chipped teeth, aspiration, introduction of infection, tube dislodgement, airway obstruction, pneumothorax, equipment failure, hypoxia, hypotension and arrhythmias. Emergency equipment, including that used for difficult airway management, must be available. In addition, post-intubation auscultation is not advisable due to the challenges with PPE and the risk of cross-contamination. Confirmation of tracheal tube placement should be assessed by the intubator viewing the ETT passing through the vocal cords, an appropriate capnography trace displayed on the monitor, chest movements visualized and a chest radiograph (CXR) performed to confirm the appropriate position [3].

Once intubated any 'necessary' disconnection (e.g. when connecting the patient to the critical care ventilator from a transport ventilator) in the ventilation circuit should be preceded by clamping the ETT until they are reconnected and ventilation established. This should take no longer than 5 s. ETT connections must be secure to prevent disconnection; in COVID-19 patients, this may involve using tape to prevent accidental disconnection. In addition, a closed suction (Picture 8.1) catheter should be used to prevent disconnection

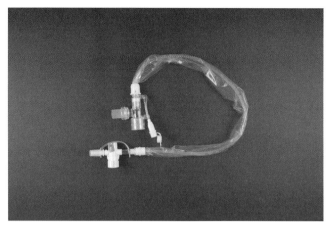

PICTURE 8.1   Closed suction catheter.

of the ventilator circuit for suctioning. This prevents hypoxia, loss of positive end-expiratory pressure (PEEP) and reduces the risk of aerosolization. Manual ventilation (also termed 'hand bagging') should be avoided due to concerns regarding aersolization and increased risk of infection [6].

The grade of intubation is used to describe the laryngeal view during laryngoscopy and to determine how difficult it is to intubate a patient. The Cormack–Lehane or Mallampati classification is the most commonly used [9], it is routinely documented and reported during hand over in case reintubation is required [10]. Ongoing care of an ETT includes noting the ETT position at the teeth or lips and checking ties are secured using ETT tape ties or commercially available tube ties such as Anchor Fast or Thomas Tube Holders. ETT cuff pressure using a manometer (Picture 8.2) should be recorded every 2–4 h, with the aim of 25–30 mmHg. Specific information handed over at each shift may include date of ETT insertion, grade (difficulty) of intubation, size of ETT, position at teeth, any signs of pressure damage from the tie, last time suctioning performed, quantity and description of secretions removed either by suctioning or aspiration of the ETT subglottic port.

Invasive ventilation

Invasive ventilation has evolved significantly since the early positive-pressure ventilators developed in the 1940s and the iron lung negative-pressure ventilators used in the polio outbreak [11]. Invasive ventilators today are now in the fourth generation of technology and allow for a range of modes [12]. Invasive ventilation assists with the movement of gases (air) into and out of the patient's lungs, while minimizing the effort of breathing (Diagram 8.1). Positive-pressure ventilation is delivered via an endotracheal or tracheostomy tube. Ventilatory

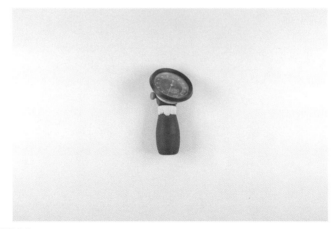

PICTURE 8.2   Manometer for measuring endotracheal and tracheostomy tube cuff pressures.

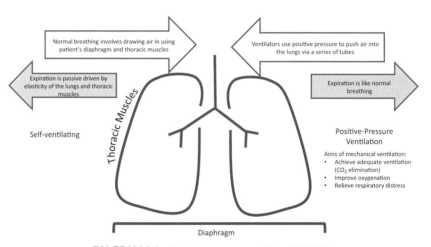

DIAGRAM 8.1   Positive-pressure ventilation [3,13,32].

support includes controlled or mandatory modes, spontaneous modes or a combination of the two [13].

As invasive modes of ventilation vary between manufacturers, each critical care unit will have their own preferences for combinations of ventilation strategies. Due to the increased demands for ventilators during the COVID-19 pandemic, hospitals may procure ventilators at short notice, that are not normally used within their critical care units, these in extremis may also include anaesthetic machines [14]. This is a cause for concern, as nurses may not have had the appropriate training, supervision, and experience of using these ventilators, which can adversely impact on patient safety [15].

Commonly used modes include synchronized intermittent mandatory ventilation (SIMV), pressure support (PS), positive end-expiratory pressure (PEEP) and continuous positive airway pressure (CPAP). High-frequency jet ventilation (HFJV), high-frequency oscillatory ventilation (HFOV) and extracorporeal membrane oxygenation (ECMO) are advanced methods of invasive ventilation and oxygenation, detailed descriptions of which are beyond the scope of this chapter. ECMO is a highly specialized procedure undertaken in tertiary referral centres. It involves completely resting the lungs and is used where standard ventilation methods have failed [3]. It must be noted that while ECMO can have a role specifically for severe COVID-19 patients who meet a specific requirement, the availability of ECMO beds is likely to exceed capacity and therefore it will only be available for a small proportion of patients.

SIMV delivers a predetermined respiratory rate, and either a predetermined tidal volume (volume controlled) or pressure (pressure controlled). The patient is still able to take additional breaths, and these may be supported by pressure support. Pressure support, also called assisted spontaneous breathing (ASB), is a spontaneous mode in which the patient triggers a breath and is supported by a preset pressure. This mode of ventilation can be used as a weaning method, as the level of support can be reduced as the patient becomes more alert, and is able to breathe effectively [13]. Invasive ventilation can cause weakened lung muscles and the underlying illness and sedation can affect weaning from ventilation. In addition, a ventilator has a series of valves, ventilator tubing and the ETT, which is a fraction of the patient's normal airway size. Therefore, breathing on a ventilator is often referred to as breathing through a straw, and PS allows for spontaneous breathing and compensation of the ventilator circuit resistance [3,13].

PEEP maintains airway pressure above atmospheric pressure during the expiratory phase. Arterial blood oxygenation is improved by preventing alveolar collapse during expiration and re-recruiting collapsed alveoli. This technique maintains or increases functional residual capacity (FRC) and improves diffusion throughout the lungs [13]. Usually PEEP will be at least $5\,cmH_2O$. This may need to be increased to recruit collapsed alveoli, from reduced surfactant, atelectasis, sputum retention and tracheal suctioning [3]. Continuous positive airway pressure (CPAP) is similar to PEEP but used when the patient is self-ventilating [13].

Volume control and pressure control

The oxygen/air (gas) mixture can be delivered to a patient either at a predetermined volume or pressure. Volume control (VC) delivers a preset tidal volume, however, the pressure the machine delivers is not controlled. This can result in high airway pressures causing barotrauma, pneumothorax and other complications. Pressure control (PC) delivers a predetermined inflation pressure resulting in varying tidal volumes and a reduction in the risk of complications, and is the preferred mode for most COVID-19 patients, especially those with acute lung injury (ALI) or acute respiratory distress syndrome (ARDS). A disadvantage of using PC is the possibility of a patient not receiving an adequate tidal volume which may lead to hypercarbia and underventilation [3,4,13].

To trigger or initiate a breath in a patient breathing spontaneously, the ventilator needs to sense the correct time for inspiration. Three methods are used: pressure sensing, volume/flow sensing or neutrally adjusted ventilator assist (NAVA). **Pressure sensing** involves the ventilator sensing a drop in the ventilator circuit as the patient tries to breathe. However, the length of ventilator tubing and effort required to trigger a breath may be too difficult and uncomfortable for many patients, and may result in the patient failing to synchronize with the ventilator. **Volume/flow sensing** provides constant gas throughout the ventilator circuit and allows for gas returning to the ventilator to be compared to the amount flowing out. When a change is detected, a breath is triggered. **NAVA** is a specialist mode of ventilation not commonly used, which involves sensing the electrical activity of the diaphragm via an oesophageal electrode in order to trigger inspiration [3,13].

Cycling refers to how the ventilator switches from inspiration to expiration and there are four types. Firstly, **time cycling** involves the inspiratory phase lasting for a fixed period of time; the ventilator then automatically switches to expiration. Secondly, **volume cycling** is where, once the present tidal volume has been reached, the ventilator switches to expiration. Thirdly, **pressure cycling** is when the preset inspiratory level is reached and the ventilator switches to expiration. Finally, **flow cycling** allows for the inspiratory phase to switch when the flow falls below a certain level, for example, once the breath is completed.

Assembly of the ventilator

Prior to commencing invasive ventilation, the critical care team needs to be aware of the patient's normal lung function whenever possible so that parameters can be set to deliver appropriate and realistic targets for oxygenation [3]. Ventilators need to be assembled as per the manufacturer guidance, and require both oxygen and gas sources and a continuous power supply, ideally with generator back-up. In addition, for COVID-19, ventilator filters must be validated against the passage of a variety of viral and bacterial species [6].

Nurses working at the bedside must be able to detect complications due to invasive ventilation (Table 8.1). These may include airway complications such as upper airway damage, laryngotracheal stenosis, fistula formation, intubation of the right main bronchus and ETT blockage or displacement, for example, during coughing or self-extubation. Breathing complications include ventilator disconnection, ventilator-associated pneumonia (VAP), barotrauma due to excessive airway pressures, volutrauma damage due to excessive lung volumes, atelectasis, and oxygen toxicity due to persistent high oxygen concentrations. Pressure on the ventilator tubing includes biting on the ETT, sputum

TABLE 8.1 Potential complications of invasive ventilation [3,13].

Airway	Upper airway damage
	Laryngotracheal stenosis and fistula formation
	Intubation of the right main bronchus
	Unplanned extubation
Breathing	Ventilator-associated pneumonia (VAP)
	Barotrauma (excessive airway pressures)
	Volutrauma (damage from excessive lung volumes)
	Atelectasis
	Oxygen toxicity due to persistent high oxygen concentrations
	Complications associated with suctioning, manually ventilating and inadequate humidification
	Obstruction, e.g., pressure on the ventilator tubing, biting on the ETT, sputum plugs blocking the ETT or TT, bronchospasm
	Pneumothorax can be simple or life threatening, resulting in a tension pneumothorax
Circulation	Increased intrathoracic pressure causing reduced venous return resulting in reduced blood pressure and increased right ventricular workload
	Use of sedation and analgesic drugs causes hypotension
	Fluid retention causing gastrointestinal disturbances and gastric distension
	Acute ulceration of the gastric and bowel mucosa
Disability (neurological)	Discomfort (coughing, gagging or biting on ETT)
	Raised intracranial pressure due to suctioning
	Complications of over/under-sedating patients
	Prolonged use of sedation may lead to delirium, polyneuropathy
Exposure, environmental	Pressure damage to the mouth and neck due to ETT ties
	Reduced mobility and muscle wastage
	Equipment problems: Power and oxygen failures. Emergency equipment must always be available at the bedside and during transfer in case of equipment failure

plugs blocking the ETT or TT, bronchospasm, and pneumothorax (simple or life threatening). Circulatory complications include increased intrathoracic pressure. This causes reduced venous return, and leads to reduced blood pressure and increased right ventricular workload. Sedation and analgesic drugs can cause hypotension, while fluid retention can cause gastrointestinal disturbances and gastric distension. Neurological problems include discomfort due to coughing, gagging or biting on ETT. Complications of over-, or under-, sedating patients, and/or prolonged use of sedation can cause delirium and polyneuropathy. Long-term effects of delirium include post-traumatic stress disorder (PTSD), delayed discharge and prolonged recovery. Other difficulties associated with invasive ventilation include pressure damage to the mouth, lips and neck due to ETT ties. In addition, for patients requiring prolonged ventilation, complex weaning impacts on mobility, resulting in muscle wastage that compounds delayed recovery [3,4,6,13]. In consequence, nurses must be acutely aware of, recognize and respond to the wider issues associated with patients requiring invasive ventilation.

The increasing numbers of severe COVID-19 patients requiring invasive ventilation is likely to place a critical demand on oxygen supplies, which may lead to supply failure [6]. In addition, increasing demand for ventilators and different types of ventilators being used in practice may lead to a critical lack of consumables, compromising patient safety.

Care of a patient requiring invasive ventilation

Patients requiring invasive ventilation need to be closely observed and continuously monitored. Although ventilators have alarms, they do not replace close observation of the patient and immediate access to a registered nurse, experienced and competent in caring for a ventilated patient [16] (Table 8.2). The monitoring of ventilated patients must include ECG, pulse oximetry and end tidal carbon dioxide ($EtCO_2$). Ventilator observations include mode of ventilation, respiratory rate (set/actual), fraction of inspired oxygen (FiO_2), airway pressures, tidal volumes, minute volume and inspiratory:expiratory (I:E) ratio. Common ventilator settings are outlined in Table 8.3. Vital signs and ventilator observations must be recorded frequently. The standard practice is to perform this hourly or if there is a change in patient condition or ventilator settings (Table 8.4). During the COVID-19 pandemic, with a diluted skill mix and less availability of critical care trained staff, the frequency of ventilator observations may be decreased, which is a cause for concern as it may lead to failure to recognize deterioration and complications early, delaying response and reducing the opportunity for patient improvement (Diagram 8.2).

Arterial blood gases (ABGs) are used to assess oxygenation and to guide clinical decision-making. These should not be performed routinely, but in response to the patient's condition or changes in treatment or ventilator settings. Sedation and pain should be assessed using validated tools such as the Richmond Agitation and Sedation Scale (RASS) and the Critical Care Pain Observation Tool (CCPOT). In consequence, nurses must be able to monitor, analyse, interpret and respond to a range of information, taking appropriate action when abnormal parameters have been identified [13,16].

Ventilator-associated pneumonia

Ventilator-associated pneumonia (VAP) has no universal, internationally agreed definition [17]. However, it is a type of pneumonia that occurs 48–72 h after intubation in invasively ventilated patients. VAP can be broadly categorized as possible or probable VAP. **Possible VAP** is indicated if there

TABLE 8.2 Typical ventilator settings for an average adult (75 kg) [28].

The following is a guide to possible ventilator settings. Patients must be individually assessed for appropriate ventilation settings.

Respiratory rate	14–16 breaths per minute
Tidal volumes	6–8 mL/kg (based on ideal body weight) for normal lungs
I:E ratio	1:2
PEEP	5 cmH$_2$O 8–10 cmH$_2$O may be indicated in pulmonary oedema or ARDS
FiO$_2$	Start high and reduce depending on SaO$_2$
Airway pressures	Plateau pressure is the highest level of pressure applied to the airway and lungs during inspiration. Measured in cmH$_2$O, with a target of <30 cmH$_2$O Peak pressure <35 cmH$_2$O

Ventilator settings tend to be changed one at a time, and incrementally. The change should be reassessed within 1–2 h.
Ventilator settings must only be changed by staff who have been assessed as competent.

TABLE 8.3 Potential ventilator alarms and causes [13,28].

High-pressure alarm	• Decreased lung compliance, e.g., pneumonia, atelectasis • Kink in the ETT • Obstruction of the ventilator tubing • Secretions in the airway or obstruction of the ETT • Bronchospasm/coughing • Biting on the tube • Movement of ETT into the right bronchus • Excessive tidal volumes being set • Patient–ventilator asynchrony
Low-pressure alarm	• Ventilator disconnection • ETT leak, e.g., ETT position changed or cuff leak
Apnoea	• Patient not breathing within a preset timeframe

are purulent secretions or positive microbiology cultures from the respiratory tract. Conversely, **probable VAP** is evidenced by purulent secretions and positive microbiology cultures from the respiratory tract and/or pleural fluid, lung histopathology or other specific diagnostic tests. Possible causes of VAP include aspiration during intubation, vomiting a feed, multiple intubations, the patient is immune compromised, has COPD, ARDS, chronic disease or

TABLE 8.4 Nursing considerations.

Safety considerations:
- Emergency oxygen and suction available at bed space
- Bag, valve mask and/or Water's circuit at bedside
- Appropriately sized suction catheters
- Being aware of different alarms and responding
- Alarm limits checked and on
- Do not modify, silence any settings on the ventilator unless trained and deemed competent to do so
- Never leave an intubated and ventilated patient unattended
- Respond to any ventilator or monitor alarms immediately
- Avoid ventilator disconnection

Endotracheal care:
- Confirm position of ETT at lips and chest ties are secure. If the ETT needs to be resecured, this is a two-person technique. Devices include:
  - Tapes. These should be changed once a shift or when wet, lose or dirty
  - Special devices, e.g., Anchor Fast, Thomas Tube holders
- Check ETT cuff pressure a minimum of every 4 h
- Closed suction catheters should be changed every 72 h or as per local guidelines. ETT should be clamped when disconnecting the patient from the ventilator and the ventilator paused to prevent aerosolization of droplets
- When indicated tracheal suction pressures should be no more than 20 kPa. Observe type and amount of secretions
- Rigid suction catheter should be used for oral suctioning

Vital signs monitoring:
- Continuous ECG monitoring
- Continuous pulse oximetry
- Continuous end tidal carbon dioxide monitoring. Good waveform suggests there is good ventilation and a patent airway
- Blood pressure monitoring (arterial line will allow for arterial blood gas analysis as indicated)

Ventilator observations:
- Mode of ventilation.
- Respiratory rate (set/actual)
- FiO_2
- Tidal volumes
- Minute volume
- IE ratio
- Plateau pressure
- Peak pressure

Ongoing care

- Hourly sedation scoring using validated scoring tool
- Hourly pain assessment using validated scoring tool
- Assess for delirium using a validated scoring tool, e.g., CAM-ICU
- Ventilator settings tend to be changed one at a time, and incrementally. The change should be reassessed within 1–2 h
- Silence alarms before disconnecting. Clamp ETT as per local policy
- Eye care
- Pressure area assessment and care
- Regular repositioning

- Communication tools, e.g., alphabet boards
- Communication with significant others
- Follow the ventilator care bundle
- ABG 4-hourly or as indicated
- Chest physiotherapy is indicated in patients who are unable to independently clear their secretions, to help reverse atelectasis and reduce work of breathing
- Report any abnormal parameters/traces immediately. This includes any change in $EtCO_2$ traces, PaO_2 <8, $PaCO_2$ >6.5, pH < 7.25, lactate >2 and/or potassium >5.5 mmol/L

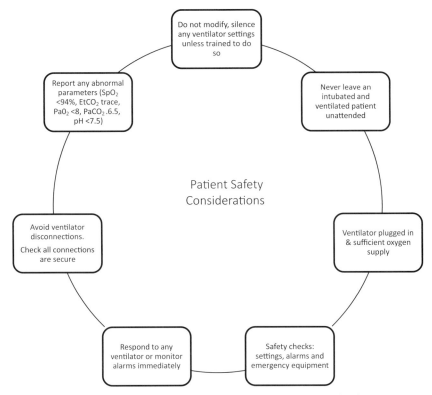

DIAGRAM 8.2   Safety considerations when nursing a ventilated patient.

has been recently hospitalized [17]. Hellyer et al. [18] argue that VAP is a major source of increased prolonged illness and death, and increased length of ICU and hospital stay and costs.

Signs of VAP may be identified when performing a respiratory assessment and include signs of sepsis and/or high or low leukocytes and other inflammatory markers, for example, C-reactive protein. Patients frequently present with increased amounts of sputum, changes in consistency (thick or purulent) and colour (yellow, green). Percussion of the chest may reveal dullness over the infected area, requiring increasing ventilatory support and oxygen requirements [3]. Preventative strategies include the use of the ventilator care bundle (VCB). This includes maintaining a bed elevation of >30 degrees, deep vein thrombosis (DVT) prophylaxis, peptic ulcer prophylaxis, managing sedation effectively (this includes a daily sedation hold as appropriate), oral care with chlorhexidine and subglottic aspiration of the ET tube (Picture 8.3). Each intervention needs to have a proven evidence base and the VCB changes as the evidence evolves [19–21].

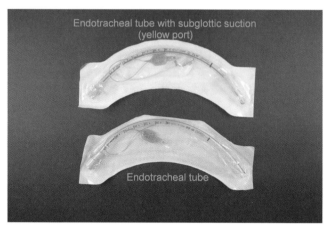

PICTURE 8.3 Endotracheal tube with or without subglottic suction port.

Humidification

Patients with an ETT or TT bypass the normal processes of cleaning, humidifying and warming that take place in the upper respiratory tract [3]. Therefore, gases delivered by invasive or non-invasive ventilation need to be clean, humidified and warm. To prevent pathogens and foreign bodies entering the patient's body, invasive ventilators have humidification and warming systems in the circuit.

Humidification can either be active or passive. Active humidification may be used in long-term ventilation, and is achieved by passing gas through an external, heated water bath chamber (wet circuit). The technique includes a heated source, water chamber or humidification chamber, temperature control unit and gas/liquid interface [22]. The heat source warms distilled water, producing water vapour. Gas collects the water vapour as it passes through the chamber, before reaching the patient. Heated humidification circuits can be used with or without a heated wire breathing circuit, which reduces the condensation in the ventilator circuit and reduces the risk of complications, for example, pooling of water in the inlet limb of the ventilator circuit tubing and thermal injury to the patient [22].

Passive humidification may be appropriate in short-term ventilation (usually less than 3 days) for example for postoperative patients, using a heat and moisture exchange (HME) filter, fitted into the ventilator circuit [3,22]. An HME requires the moisture and heat from the patients expired breath to be recycled through a filter system. This type of humidification is termed a 'dry circuit'. The HME should be placed as close to the patient as possible, often placed between the catheter mount and the patient's ETT. The frequency of changing HMEs is determined by local infection prevention and control guidelines, but any manipulation of the ventilator circuit may result in contamination [22].

Severe COVID-19 patients requiring invasive ventilation are at risk of the build-up of secretions and obstruction of ETT (plugging), particularly when using dry humidification. When using a wet circuit, the filters can represent an airflow obstruction when saturated, therefore regular assessment and replacement are required. However, when using both a dry and wet humidification system simultaneously, the 'wet' humidification increases the risk of breaking of the ventilator circuit due to the build-up of fluid in the ventilator tubing and regular changing of HMEs [7]. In consequence, all filters including HMEs should be checked regularly for water saturation, a maximum of 12-hourly, and routinely changed as indicated, but left no longer than 24 h or as per the manufacturer's guidelines.

Improving oxygenation in COVID-19 patients

Patients with severe COVID-19 infection commonly develop ARDS [23]. The Berlin definition is used to categorize the severity of ARDS [24]. For severe COVID-19 patients who develop ARDS, management includes using lung protection strategies (low-volume, low-pressure ventilation): tidal volume 6 mL/kg and plateau airway pressure <30 cmH$_2$O. Early evidence suggests pressures may need to be lower than previously recommended [25]. There needs to be pre-oxygenation of patients prior to any intervention, for example, suctioning to prevent prolonged periods of desaturation.

The use of nitric oxide or nebulized prostacyclin if using a wet circuit has been noted to improve vasodilation and thus improve oxygenation and reduce airway pressures [25]. PEEP may be used to recruit collapsed alveoli; however, high PEEP should be avoided. Recruitment manoeuvres are used to improve oxygenation by providing brief inspiratory flow cycles to maximum plateau pressure and inflating collapsed alveoli. Recruitment manoeuvres tend to be used as a rescue therapy in severe refractory hypoxia or following accidental disconnection from the ventilator. The procedure remains controversial in routine care, as it provides a temporary increase in oxygenation which is not sustained, and therefore must only be performed by an experienced practitioner [26,27].

To improve oxygenation, prone positioning should be considered early and, if necessary, repeated several times until oxygenation improves. Prone positioning involves placing an invasively ventilated patient face down to improve oxygenation–ventilation–perfusion. Recently, intensive care experience has shown a beneficial response to prone position use by COVID-19 patients not yet requiring invasive ventilation [27]. Early recommendations are that proning patients on admission to ICU during the early phase of their disease may be beneficial and avoid more aggressive ventilation strategies. It can be used irrespective of the PF ratio [25].

Neuromuscular blocking agents may be required to maintain gaseous exchange, this reduces extrapulmonary resistance and ventilatory desynchrony which in turn results in improved oxygenation. Paralysis of the diaphragm allows for metabolic rest, reduced oxygen consumption and invasive control of breathing mechanics [26]. Neuromuscular blockage may be required in patients with ARDS as this allows for less PEEP to maintain oxygenation, and reduced mortality.

A patient's haemodynamic status may impact on ventilation, for example, invasive ventilation increases the intrathoracic pressure and may result in reduced cardiac preload with venous return reduced. Intrathoracic pressure may increase during suctioning, positioning and when using PEEP [26]. A patient's pre-existing cardiac history may impact on ventilation, for example, in a patient with an impaired cardiac ejection fraction, it may impact on weaning. In consequence, perfusion as well as oxygenation need to be considered as they are interlinked and interdependent. Adequate perfusion and blood flow to the tissues are required to promote oxygenation [26].

Early mobilization of mechanically ventilated patients

Patients requiring mechanical ventilation may become immobilized, which leads to muscle loss and weakness of both the diaphragm and skeletal muscles [12]. Neuromyopathies may occur in patients who have sepsis, multiorgan failure or prolonged ventilation. Early passive and active mobility activities have been designed to reduce weakness by maintaining or restoring a patient's mobility and independence. Types of passive and active early mobilization activities used are outlined in Table 8.5. The choice of activity depends on the patient's ability to participate in activities and the resources available, for example, special chairs, manual handling devices such as sliding boards and hoists [12].

Prior to undertaking any early mobilization activities, the patient must be assessed, to ascertain that they have the requisite physiological reserve to complete the level of activity. This assessment which guides the frequency, timing and type of activity is variable, and needs to be agreed by the critical care team and evaluated daily. Barriers to early mobilization include the use of sedation,

---

TABLE 8.5 Passive and active mobilization activities [12].

Passive mobilization activities:	Active mobilization activities:
• Supported range of motion	• Participating in turning in bed
• Stretching	• In-bed exercises, e.g., weights or cycling
• Turning and repositioning in bed	• Inspiratory muscle training/breathing exercises
• Tilt-able therapy	• Sitting and/or standing balance exercises at the side of the bed
• Speciality beds	
• Passive cycle ergometer	• Transferring from bed to chair
• Neuromuscular electrical stimulation	• Assisted ambulation
	• Independent ambulation

presence of an ETT, respiratory and cardiovascular instability and neurological impairment [12].

Potential adverse events that can occur during early mobilization include accidental extubation, hyper- and hypotension, oxygen desaturation, arrhythmias and removal of NG tubes and lines, for example, arterial [12]. To prevent these and improve effectiveness, a multidisciplinary approach to patient care including input from nurses, physiotherapists, dieticians and doctors must be used, in conjunction with agreed inclusion and exclusion criteria and protocols. Other considerations include fall prevention assessment and risk assessment, delirium assessment and management, sedation guidelines, and nutrition and sleep hygiene guidelines.

Weaning from invasive ventilation

Weaning off invasive ventilation is the process used to assist an individual to breathe unaided. The process is complex and may take days, weeks or months. The weaning plan should be individualized and commenced once the patient is placed on an invasive ventilator. It includes correcting the cause of the respiratory failure, maintaining muscle strength, maintaining adequate nutritional support and psychological preparation [13].

The speed at which a patient may be weaned will be determined by the factors outlined above and may be short or long term. Principles of weaning include a pre-weaning assessment and the development of a multidisciplinary weaning plan [13]. Patients ventilated for less than 3 days may be able to be weaned faster (short term) than those who have been ventilated for a longer period. Long-term weaning is more complex and follows the same principles as short-term weaning, however, the process is more gradual and involves a multidisciplinary approach. In addition, a tracheostomy may be performed to assist with weaning. Prolonged weaning can have a negative psychological effect on the patient and their families. It is therefore important to explain the stages in the weaning plan and each stage [3,13]

The pre-weaning assessment should be undertaken each day by the critical care team and appropriate parameters set relating to oxygenation and weaning. Individualized parameters should be set by the team to facilitate weaning. Patients can quickly become dependent on invasive ventilation, and the weaning plan allows a gradual reintroduction to normal breathing. The longer the patient has been ventilated, the more complex a weaning plan may be required. Weaning whilst on high concentrations of oxygen is not recommended.

The weaning phase and plan vary between patients and are determined by the pre-weaning assessment. Weaning plans should be started in the morning or early afternoon. Patients should not be weaned overnight, but allowed to rest. Weaning involves stopping all or most sedation and assessing the patient, explaining the procedure to the patient, suctioning the airway as indicated, continuing monitoring and assessment, sitting the patient upright to maximize chest expansion, a Glasgow Coma Scale >8, and a cough reflex. The patient must be on a spontaneous mode of ventilation with a low PEEP and PS, be able to protect their own airway, and a rescue plan must be agreed in case the procedure fails. An ABG may be taken after 20–30 min of spontaneous breathing. If within normal parameters, and following review from the intensivist, it may be appropriate to consider extubation. It must be noted that weaning may take several days or weeks, using an individualized assessment and plan.

Extubation involves the removal of an ETT when the patient is stable and no longer requires an artificial airway. Planned extubations should take place during the daytime when additional staff, and suitably trained or skilled staff who can intubate, are available. The patient should be extubated early so that their progress can be monitored and, if any additional input is needed, it can be identified early. Following intubation, the patient should be monitored and reassessed as indicated. Indications for reintubation include uncoordinated respiratory function, exhaustion, agitation and poor oxygenation [13]. The individual rescue plan for a patient must be agreed by the critical care team and should include identifying if it would be appropriate to reintubate. If necessary, non-invasive ventilation (NIV) may be used to prevent reintubation. However, it must be noted that in COVID-19 cases, evidence suggests reintubation rates within 24–48 h are higher than expected (up to 60%). These patients can have severe upper airway swelling and the use of dexamethasone and nebulized adrenaline can be used. In consequence, delaying initial extubation for longer may prevent reintubation when the need for access to specialist staff is immediately required [25].

Unplanned extubation is a serious complication as the patient may not be ready, with the result that emergency reintubation may be required (Table 8.6).

TABLE 8.6 Emergency situations [13].

Unplanned extubation
- This is an emergency situation. Immediately call for help/emergency buzzer
- Assemble emergency intubation equipment
- Assess patient:
  - Self-ventilating: non-rebreath mask 15 L/min
  - Unconscious: Insert oropharyngeal airway, ventilate using bag, valve mask (15 L/min). Prepare for reintubation
  - Check NG feed has been stopped and NG tube aspirated

ETT cuff leak
- Signs of ETT cuff leak: gurgling sounds
- Assess patient:
  - Check cuff pressure with a manometer
  - Inflate cuff and recheck cuff pressure
  - If no improvement – call for help/inform doctors
  - Document actions

There is evidence to suggest that in patients who require reintubation, it may result in setbacks in their recovery and should be avoided. Reasons for unplanned extubation include the patient being awake and pulling at the ETT tube or the tube becoming dislodged during patient care, for example, during repositioning. There is a possibility of increased self-extubation due to limited staff and patients who are over-sedated. In the event of an unplanned extubation, it should be regarded as an emergency, the nurse must immediately assess the patient (ABCDE approach) and call for help. If necessary, airway management procedures should be initiated and the patient oxygenated. If they are self-ventilating, high-flow oxygen should be started. If the patient is apnoeic then an appropriately sized oropharyngeal airway should be inserted and ventilation commenced using a bag, valve mask and a two-person technique.

Nursing care of a suspected or confirmed COVID-19 patient with a tracheostomy

A tracheostomy tube (TT) requires a surgical opening in the anterior wall of the trachea and the insertion of the tube. In critical care, tracheostomies may be carried out in patients who require prolonged mechanical ventilation. As a result of COVID-19 the role of tracheostomy to support weaning is unclear, given this is AGP and care is being provided in the context of a resource-limited, overwhelmed system. However, with increasing numbers of patients requiring mechanical ventilation, tracheostomy may be appropriate in some patients. The benefits may include lower risk of laryngeal injury compared to prolonged intubation, improved comfort for the patient, assisting with weaning from mechanical ventilation, improved tracheal secretion removal, enhanced patient communication and decreased sedation requirements. In the event of a patient requiring a tracheostomy, nursing care includes maintaining a patent airway and checking the TT dressing is clean and intact (Table 8.7). TT tubes are secured using Velcro straps (Picture 8.4).

Critically ill patients who require a tracheostomy (percutaneous or surgical) should have them performed electively, by the most skilled practitioner, so that the procedure is safe, accurate and swift [29]. If the procedure is to be done as a percutaneous tracheostomy in critical care, only essential staff should be at the bedside during the procedure, wearing full PPE (including a FFP3 mask and eye/face protection) and with a runner outside. The procedure must be performed as an aseptic procedure; therefore a sterile disposable gown and sterile gloves must be worn over PPE during the procedure.

When performing routine tracheostomy care, for example changing a tracheostomy inner tube (Picture 8.5) or aspirating the subglottic port of the tracheostomy (Picture 8.6), due to the risks from secretions and coughing, PPE must be worn, including a mask (FFP3 or surgical mask with integrated visor), full face shield/visor, and a fluid-resistant disposable gown. If a non-fluid-resistant gown is used a disposable plastic apron must be worn underneath [29,30].

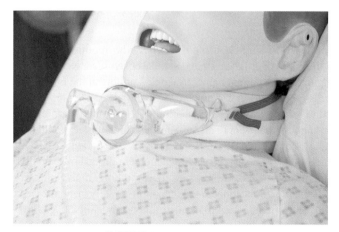

PICTURE 8.4 Tracheostomy.

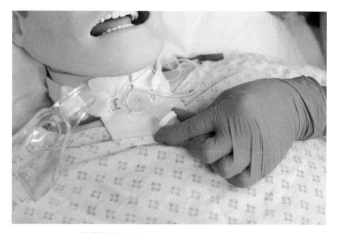

PICTURE 8.5 Tracheostomy inner tube.

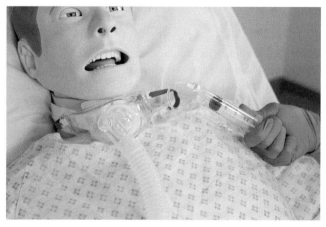

PICTURE 8.6 Aspirating subglottic port of tracheostomy.

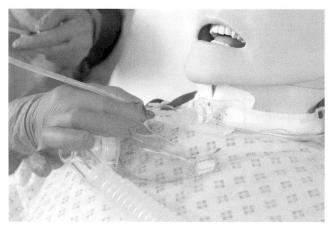

PICTURE 8.7   Suctioning a tracheostomy tube.

Tracheostomy tube cuffs must remain inflated to reduce the risk of transmission. Cuff pressures using a manometer should be checked every 2–4 h, aiming for a pressure of 25–30 mmHg. Cuffed non-fenestrated tracheostomy tubes should be used to avoid aerosolizing the virus, therefore, this may delay the decannulation process. If the patient is ventilated, an HME (heat and moisture exchanger) should be placed on the tracheostomy to reduce the viral spread if the ventilator tubing becomes disconnected. If disconnection is necessary, for example to connect to a transport ventilator, the disconnection should be distal to the HME. In addition, a closed suction system should be used to prevent the risk of disconnection, loss of oxygen and PEEP and reduce viral spread [29,30].

In non-ventilated tracheostomy patients with suspected or confirmed COVID-19, staff must wear full PPE including an FFP3 mask and goggles as per local and national guidelines, as coughing and open suctioning are classed as an AGP (Picture 8.7). Suctioning and inner cannula care are high-risk airway interventions, therefore, staff must be appropriately trained in tracheostomy care and recognizing and responding to tracheostomy emergencies [31]. Supplementary oxygen may be required and should be delivered via a tracheostomy mask (Picture 8.4), this may offer some protection from the immediate environmental droplet spread. Patients with a tracheostomy are likely to need open humidification, and depending on resources and local protocols this may range from a Buchanan bib, simple HME device or active warmed humidification. When the tracheostomy cuff is deflated, to minimize droplet spread a simple face mask should be applied over the patient's face [30].

Emergency tracheostomy equipment must be available at the patient's bedside at all times. Equipment includes spare-cuffed tracheostomy tubes and inner cannula (one that is the same type and size as the patient and one size smaller than the size the patient has inserted), tracheal dilators to maintain stoma opening in

TABLE 8.7 Tracheostomy care.

- Staff wearing PPE including FFP3 and goggles in accordance with local and national guidelines
- Check tracheostomy cuff pressure every 4 h using a manometer
- If possible, use a closed suction system
- Check/change inner tube every 4 h
- If tracheostomy has a subglottic port aspirate 4-hourly
- Clean inner tube using sterile water, do not use brushes
- If ventilated use continuous $EtCO_2$ monitoring to confirm tube position and early identification of complications
- Humidify oxygen if not ventilated
- Check/clean stoma site regularly
- Provide oral care every 6 h
- When using a speaking valve, always deflate the cuff first
- Consider appropriate communication strategies
- Document your actions and findings

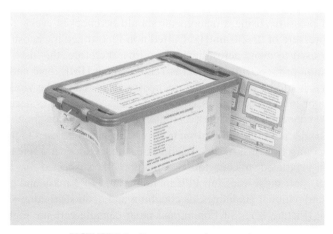

PICTURE 8.8   Emergency tracheostomy box

the event of accidental tube removal until the replacement tube is inserted, suture cutter for removal of a tube that is sutured in place, for example, when surgically inserted, sterile scissors to cut cotton tracheostomy tapes, 10 mL syringes to deflate/inflate cuffs, tracheostomy tapes and Velcro holder, tracheostomy dressing, water-soluble lubricant, cleaning swab, occlusive dressing and gauze [31].

In many settings, boxes with tamper-proof seals are used to contain all the equipment (Picture 8.8). Staff must check the tracheostomy tube sizes are correct for the patient and that the equipment has not expired. In addition, access to an oxygen supply, suction (walled or portable) and appropriately sized suction catheter must be immediately available.

Conclusion

The rapid deterioration that occurs from the nature of COVID-19 leading to tracheal intubation and the nurse's role in the management of patients with COVID-19 on invasive ventilation has been explored. The impact of COVID-19 is such that critical care nurses and their redeployed colleagues have had to face a radical change in the ways in which they care for and support ventilated patients. Additional approaches were not designed for the rapid changes in patient status or the scale of patients needing critical care. It is important that during this time of crisis, the long-term effects and impact of invasive ventilation are not overlooked. The aim of this chapter has been to enable nurses to adapt their practice to meet the current situation, while making every effort to maintain patient safety, and to protect themselves, their colleagues and peers.

References

[1] Alphonso A, Quinones M, Mishra A, et al. A study to evaluate the competency of ICU personnel in mechanical ventilation. 2004.

[2] Burns SM. Mechanical ventilation of patients with acute respiratory distress syndrome and patients requiring weaning. Crit Care Nurse 2005;25(4):14–24.

[3] Elliot ZJ, Elliot SC. An overview of mechanical ventilation in the intensive care unit. Nurs Stand 2018;32(28):41–9.

[4] Goldsworthy S. Preface. Mechanical ventilation in the critically ill patient: international nursing perspectives. 2016.

[5] Kajal K, Hazarika A, Reddy S, Jain K, Meena SC. Emergency intubation outside operating room/intensive care unit settings: are we following the recommendations for safe practice? Anaesth Essay Res 2018;12(4):865–72.

[6] NHS England. Clinical guide for the management of critical care patients during the coronavirus pandemic. 2020. Version 1.

[7] Cook TM, El–Boghdadly K, McGuire B, McNarry AF, Patel A, Higgs A. Consensus guidelines for managing the airway in patients with COVID–19. Anaesthesia 2020;75(6):785-799. https://doi.org/10.1111/anae.15054.

[8] Sorbello M, Afshari A, DeHert S. Device or target? A paradigm shift in airway management: implications for guidelines, clinical practice and teaching. Eur J Anaesthesiol 2018;35:811–4.

[9] Krage R, van Rijn C, van Groeningen D, Loer SA, Schwarte LA, Schober P. Cormack-Lehane classification revisited -. Br J Anaesth 2010;105(2):220–7.

[10] Sharma M. Grade of intubation vs Laryngoscopy CL view. Br J Anaesth 2015;115. eLetters Supplement. https://doi.org/10.1093/bja/el_12732.

[11] Kelly FE, Fong K, Hirsch N, Nolan JP. Intensive care medicine is 60 years old: the history and future of the intensive care unit. Clin Med 2014;14(4):376–9.

[12] Hruska P. Early mobilization of mechanically ventilated patients. Crit Care Nurs Clin 2016;28:413–24.

[13] Edwards S, Williams J. In: A nurse's survival guide to critical care. Elsevier; 2019. Updated.

[14] Gov.uk. Anaesthetic machines; off label use during COVID_19 pandemic. 2020. https://www.gov.uk/drug-device-alerts/anaesthetic-machines-off-label-use-during-the-covid-19-pandemic-mda-2020-01.

[15] Gilroy R. Covid-19 ventilator appeal 'pointless' without staff and other kit. Nurs Times 2020. 16 March 2020 https://www.nursingtimes.net.

[16] World Federation of Critical Care Nurses. Position statement: provision of a critical care nursing workforce. 2019. www.wfccn.org.

[17] Baid H. Patient safety: identifying and managing complications of mechanical ventilation. Crit Care Nurs Clin N Am 2016;28:451–62.

[18] Hellyer TP, Ewan V, Wilson P, et al. The intensive care society recommended bundle of interventions for the prevention of ventilator-associated pneumonia. J Intens Care Soc 2016;17(3):238-243. https://doi.org/10.1177/1751143716644461.

[19] Klompas M, Speck K, Howell MD, et al. Reappraisal of routine oral care with chlorhexidine gluconate for patients receiving mechanical ventilation. J Am Med Assoc 2014;174(5):751.

[20] Wong T, Schlichting AB, Stoltze AJ, et al. No decrease in early ventilator associated pneumonia after early use of chlorhexidine. Am J Crit Care 2016;25(2):173–7.

[21] National Institute for Health and Clinical Excellence. Technical patient safety solutions for ventilator associated pneumonia in adults. 2016. [London].

[22] Selvaraj N. Artificial humification for the mechanically ventilated patient. Nurs Stand 2010;25(8):41–6.

[23] ARDS Definition Task Force, Ranieri VM, Rubenfeld GD, Thompson BT, Ferguson ND, Caldwell E, Fan E, Camporota L, Slutsky AS. Acute respiratory distress syndrome: the Berlin Definition. J Am Med Assoc 2012;307(23):2526–33. PMID: 22797452.

[24] Life in the Fast Lane. Acute respiratory distress Syndrome definitions. 2020. https://litfl.com/acute-respiratory-distress-syndrome-definitions/.

[25] Intensive Care Society. COVID-19: a synthesis of clinical experience in UK intensive care settings. 2020. London Barton et al. 2016.

[26] Poston JT, Patel BK, Davis AM. Management of critically ill adults with COVID-19. JAMA 2020;26. https://doi.org/10.1001/jama.2020.4914.

[27] Bamford P, Bentley A, Dean J, Whitmore D, Wilson-Baig N. ICS guidance for prone positioning of the conscious COVID patient 2020. London: Intensive Care Society; 2020.

[28] Intensive Care Foundation. Handbook of mechanical ventilation – a user's guide. 2015. [London].

[29] ENT UK. Tracheostomy guidance during the COVID-19 pandemic. 2020. https://www.entuk.org/tracheostomy-guidance-during-covid-19-pandemic.

[30] National Tracheostomy Safety Project. NTSP considerations for tracheostomy in the Covid-19 outbreak. 2020. www.trachesotmy.org.uk.

[31] Billington J, Luckett A. Care of the critically ill patient with a tracheostomy. Nurs Stand 2019. https://doi.org/10.7748/ns.2019.e11297.

[32] What would Florence do? New to ITU ventilation basics: a very basic overview of invasive ventilation. 2020. www.whatwouldflorencedo.com.

Chapter 9

Acute respiratory distress syndrome and the prone position in COVID-19

Rosaleeta Reece-Anthony, Chris Carter, Grace Lao, Joy Notter

Chapter Outline

COVID-19 causes acute respiratory failure, with an estimated 10% of patients developing acute respiratory distress syndrome (ARDS), which is associated with a high mortality of approximately 30%–40% despite advanced treatment [1]. As a consequence, the rapid increase in the need for critical care has resulted in many hospitals, regions and countries coming close to, or being overwhelmed by, an unprecedented number of patients. As knowledge and understanding of this new Coronavirus advances, effective treatment measures have been increasingly identified. One of these, prone positioning, was not commonly used in critical care units prior to the COVID-19 pandemic [2–4], and has revolutionized the treatment of both ventilated and non-ventilated patients. However, its reintroduction has confirmed that it should not be seen as a standalone measure. To be effective, it needs to be a core component of a series of structured interventions. This chapter explores the use of the prone position in ARDS arising from COVID-19.

Respiratory failure

COVID-19 disease progression may range from mild to severe [5]. High numbers of hospitalized patients develop respiratory symptoms, with a reported

COVID-19: A Critical Care Textbook. https://doi.org/10.1016/B978-0-7020-8383-9.00009-9

121

incidence of over 80% of patients needing oxygen therapy [6,7]. Patients with increasingly severe COVID-19 symptoms may go on to develop acute respiratory failure and subsequently ARDS. It should be noted that these patients may not follow the typical ARDS disease trajectory [8]. In the literature, this has been described by the term 'happy hypoxaemia' or 'silent hypoxia', when an individual has profound hypoxia caused by COVID-19, but does not have the proportional signs of respiratory distress [9–11]. As a consequence, there has been a suggestion that the term CARDS (COVID-19 with ARDS) should be used instead of the traditional ARDS definition [8]. The causes of this paradox are complex and not yet fully understood, with the result that varying pathophysiological hypotheses have been proposed [8,12].

The phenotype theory hypothesis is that in severe COVID-19 disease, there is a systemic impact on the vascular endothelium, causing lung injury. Marini and Gattinoni [8] proposed that in COVID-19, Type L and Type H phenotypes cause different variants of respiratory failure (Diagram 9.1). Type L patients have a scattered ground-glass appearance on chest X-ray, with good lung compliance and tend not to be positive end expiratory pressure (PEEP) responsive. Contrastingly, individuals with Type H respiratory failure have extensive infiltrates with both atelectasis and oedema on chest X-ray, adding further complexity to disease management. These patients have a lower lung compliance and are PEEP responsive. However, Marini and Gattinoni [8] described the Type L and H phenotypes as a continuum, with some stages and characteristics overlapping. They argued that during the early phases of respiratory failure, a complex process of pulmonary vascular dysregulation occurs, which instead of causing alveolar oedema leads to hypoxaemia and a high minute volume ventilation, but they exhibit no signs of respiratory failure. As pulmonary vascular

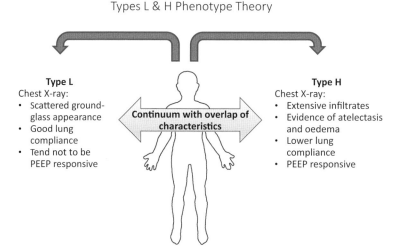

DIAGRAM 9.1 Types L and H phenotype theory. *PEEP*, positive end expiratory pressure.

dysregulation continues and extends, vasoplegia causes the lungs to become increasingly unable to regulate perfusion and maintain adequate ventilation. This exacerbates hypoxaemia and causes dead space ventilation and hypercapnia, leading to ARDS.

Jain and Doyle [12] disputed the foregoing phenotype hypothesis and argued that the Type L phenotype relates to stage 2 or 3 of COVID-19 pneumonia. They proposed a different pathophysiological process for the cause of severe hypoxia (Diagram 9.2). They suggested that the SARS-CoV-2 enters the type II alveolar epithelial cells binding to the spike protein of the ACE-2 receptor. This, in turn, leads to downregulation of the alveolar epithelium, allowing for ACE-1 to have an unregulated effect on the pulmonary capillary endothelial cells. The level of protective ACE-2-Ang-1-7-mas-R production is reduced, resulting in a harmful increase in the level of ACE-1-AngII-ATI-R. Vasoconstriction in the pulmonary epithelium is caused by endothelium-1. This causes a complex cascade effect, which results in endothelial nitric oxide being inhibited. The associated severe pulmonary vasoconstriction is unevenly distributed within the lungs, as the shunt fraction increases with increasing hypoxia and the alveolar–capillary barrier is disrupted. The flooding of proteins, fibrin, cells and fluid into the alveolar space, this causes bilateral patchy group glass opacities noted on CT scan or chest X-ray. The development of pulmonary symptoms and rapid disease progression associated with COVID-19 may be linked to 'endothelial–epithelial' interaction. Following alveolar–capillary membrane disruption, SARS-CoV-2 is able to enter the pulmonary capillary membrane via the pulmonary capillaries. The pulmonary endothelial cells become infected via the ACE-2 protein on the luminal surfaces to assume a 'proinflammatory/procoagulant' phenotype. This accelerates apoptosis of alveolar epithelial and endothelial cells and causes a cytokine storm [13].

The decision when to intubate patients remains largely subjective and based on practitioners' experience and patients' condition [14]. Mohlenkamp

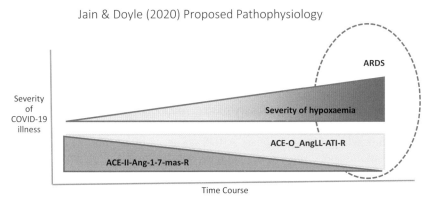

DIAGRAM 9.2 Proposed pathophysiology process in COVID-19. *ARDS*, acute respiratory distress syndrome.

et al. [15] found that 5%–15% of patients with COVID-19 require critical care and ventilatory support, with 17% of patients developing ARDS [1]. ARDS was first described in critically ill patients in 1967 by Ashbaugh et al. [16]. However, it was not until 1994 that the first clinical definition was agreed by the International American European Consensus Conference [17]. The Berlin Definition aimed to classify the severity of ARDS and to publish treatments and ventilatory strategies depending on the degree of hypoxaemia [18]. ARDS is defined using the Berlin Criteria and is based on timing, imaging, evidence of oedema and oxygenation. ARDS is defined [19] as:

> *an acute diffuse, inflammatory lung injury, leading to increased pulmonary vascular permeability, increased lung weight, and loss of aerated lung tissue … [with] hypoxemia and bilateral radiographic opacities, associated with increased venous admixture, increased physiological dead space and decreased lung compliance.*

ARDS is described as respiratory failure with an acute onset, which affects both lungs and occurs within 1 week of either a clinical insult or deterioration in respiratory symptoms. Chest imaging reveals bilateral opacities not fully explained by effusions, lung collapse and nodules. Respiratory failure is not explained by cardiac failure and fluid overload and oxygenation:

- Mild PaO_2/FiO_2 <39.9 kPa (<300 mmHg) with PEEP or continuous positive airway pressure (CPAP) >5 cmH$_2$O
- Moderate PaO_2/FiO_2 <26.6 kPa (<200 mmHg) with PEEP >5 cmH$_2$O
- Severe PaO_2/FiO_2 <13.3 kPa (<100 mmHg) with PEEP >5 cmH$_2$O

[19–21].

Limitations with the current ARDS definition show that severity can be assessed on a single blood gas without prior standardization of ventilator settings, including PEEP, which may affect oxygenation. As a consequence, it is recommended that ventilator settings are optimized using tidal volumes of 6 mL/kg of predicted body weight and a high PEEP level [22]. Furthermore, the time from optimizing ventilator settings and assessing PaO_2/FiO_2 is deemed more clinically relevant in ARDS classification when measured 24 h after ARDS onset [22].

ARDS is an acute inflammatory lung condition, not a disease, with multi-factorial causes and no proven drug treatments. Therefore ARDS is always caused by an underlying pulmonary or extra-pulmonary condition. Pulmonary ARDS occurs when there is a direct insult to the lung damaging the alveolar epithelium, while extra-pulmonary ARDS is caused by an indirect lung injury due to inflammatory mediators damaging the vascular endothelium [23,24]. Pulmonary ARDS can be caused by bacterial, viral or fungal pneumonia, aspiration of gastric contents, inhalation contusion, pulmonary contusion and pulmonary vasculitis or near drowning. Extra-pulmonary ARDS can be triggered by non-pulmonary sepsis, non-cardiogenic shock, pancreatitis, major trauma, multiple transfusion or transfusion-related acute lung injury, severe burns or drug overdose [25,26].

The majority of patients with COVID-19 who develop ARDS meet the Berlin Criteria [27]. In patients who develop ARDS, management includes using lung protection strategies: low-volume, low-pressure ventilation. Initial ventilation strategies may include pressure-controlled modes, with tidal volumes aimed at 6 mL/kg using predicted body weight and plateau airway pressure <30 cmH$_2$O. Initial ventilator settings may include a higher respiratory rate (20/min), with PEEP. Early evidence suggests pressures may need to be lower than previously recommended [4]. Permissive hypercapnia amy be accepted as long as it does not impact on other organs. In addition, moderate hypoxaemia may be accepted, in preference to high FiO$_2$ requirements. There needs to be pre-oxygenation of patients prior to any intervention, for example, suctioning to prevent prolonged periods of desaturation.

The use of nitric oxide or nebulized prostacyclin if using a wet circuit has been noted to improve vasodilation and thus improve oxygenation and reduce airway pressures [4]. PEEP may be used to recruit collapsed alveoli; however, high PEEP should be avoided. Recruitment manoeuvres are used to improve oxygenation by providing brief inspiratory flow cycles to maximum plateau pressure and inflating collapsed alveoli. Recruitment manoeuvres tend to be used as a rescue therapy in severe refractory hypoxia or following accidental disconnection from the ventilator. The procedure remains controversial in routine care, as it provides a temporary increase in oxygenation, which is not sustained, and therefore must only be performed by an experienced practitioner [28].

For patients who do not respond and become increasingly difficult to ventilate and oxygenate, the prone position may be considered. With extracorporeal membrane oxygenation (ECMO) services being limited in many settings during a pandemic, the prone position may be used as an alternative in an attempt to improve oxygenation and optimize lung compliance [29]. Conservative use of intravenous fluids and careful fluid balance monitoring with the use of diuretics to remove excess fluid should be considered, provided it is not detrimental to other organs.

Considerations for resource-limited environments

It is accepted that identifying and applying the internationally agreed ARDS definition in a resource-limited setting may be difficult due to limited availability of resources [30]. In these situations, it may be appropriate to use the Kigali-modified ARDS definition and criteria (Table 9.1). The main difference relates to the assessment of respiratory deterioration using the SpO$_2$/FiO$_2$ calculation [30].

Prone position

The prone position involves repositioning the patient from the supine position onto their abdomen. It redistributes perfusion and improves ventilation/perfusion

TABLE 9.1 Similarities and differences between the Kigali modified acute respiratory distress syndrome (ARDS) definition and the Berlin definition of ARDS.

Kigali-modified ARDS definition	Berlin definition of ARDS
Acute onset affecting both lungs occurring within 1 week of: • Clinical insult/deterioration in respiratory symptoms	Acute onset affecting both lungs occurring within 1 week of: • Clinical insult • Deterioration in respiratory symptoms
Chest X-ray or ultrasound showing: • Bilateral opacities not fully explained by effusions • Lobar/lung collapse • Nodules	Chest imaging showing: • Bilateral opacities not fully explained by effusions • Lung collapse • Nodules
Respiratory failure not fully explained by cardiac failure or fluid overload	Respiratory failure not explained by cardiac failure and fluid overload
SpO_2/FiO_2 <315 No positive end expiratory pressure (PEEP) requirement	Mild PaO_2/FiO_2 <39.9 kPa (<300 mmHg) with PEEP or continuous positive airway pressure >5 cmH$_2$O Moderate PaO_2/FiO_2 <26.6 kPa (<200 mmHg) with PEEP >5 cmH$_2$O Severe PaO_2/FiO_2 <13.3 kPa (<100 mmHg) with PEEP >5 cmH$_2$O
[30]	[19–21]

(V/Q) matching by maximizing dorsal ventilation. This results in recruitment of the posterior lung segments, causing reverse atelectasis and improved secretion clearance [28]. The prone position was first described in the literature in 1974 as a way to improve oxygenation [31]. Since that date, research has consistently shown that oxygenation can be improved in ventilated patients with ARDS by using the prone position [32–35]. However, more recent studies have shown that the prone position improves mortality in moderate to severe ARDS if undertaken early. The position needs to be maintained for 16–18 h or more while using lung-protective strategies [36]. This is a change from traditional practice, in which the prone position was solely used for ventilated patients; however, more recently, experience has shown a beneficial response to the prone position by COVID-19 patients not yet requiring invasive ventilation [28]. Early recommendations are that proning patients on admission to ICU during the early phase of their disease may be beneficial and avoid more aggressive ventilation strategies. It can be used irrespective of the PaO_2/FiO_2 ratio [4]. Both conscious and unconscious prone position methods are described here.

Conscious prone position

Conscious patients with suspected or confirmed COVID-19 who require oxygen of >28% or basic respiratory support to achieve SaO_2 92%–96% (88%–92% if high risk of hypercapnia respiratory failure) may gain benefit from the conscious prone position. If tolerated, this position can improve oxygenation, reducing the need for non-invasive ventilation. It has been found that this can delay and/or avert the need for intubation and mechanical ventilation [7,28]. The current pandemic has also revealed that this is a simple and safe intervention that is suitable for use on general wards.

If there is an improvement in SaO_2 92%–96% (88%–92% if risk of hypercapnic respiratory failure) and no obvious distress, the prone position should continue, with a view to changing the patient's position every 1–2 h or longer if possible. When not in the prone position, the patient should be nursed in a 30–60-degree upright position. Vital signs, including oxygen saturations and early warning scores, should be monitored after every position change and oxygen titrated accordingly. If tolerated, continued timed position changes can be used. A proposed regimen includes 30 min to 2 h in the following positions: lying fully prone with the bed flat, lying on their right side with the bed flat, sitting upright 30–60 degrees, lying on left side with the bed flat, prone position again and then repeated. The position should be discontinued if there is no improvement, the patient is unable to tolerate the position, the respiratory rate is >35, and there is evidence of tiring and/or the use of accessory muscles [28]. If appropriate, the patient should be reviewed by critical care and assessment made regarding transfer into critical care.

Absolute contraindications include respiratory distress ≥35 breaths per minute, $PaCO_2$ ≥6.5, and/or accessory muscle use, the immediate need for intubation, haemodynamic instability (systolic blood pressure <90 mmHg) or arrhythmia, agitation or altered mental status and unstable spine/thoracic injury/recent abdominal surgery. Relative contraindications include facial injuries, neurological issues, morbid obesity, pregnancy (2nd/3rd trimesters) and pressure sores/ulcers [28].

To turn a conscious patient into the prone position, it is important to explain the importance of the procedure to the patient (Diagram 9.1) to provide reassurance, improve oxygenation and reduce their chance of requiring invasive ventilation. Patients should be encouraged to remain in the prone position for as long as possible, ideally up to 18 h per 24 h. Patients must be assisted into and out of the prone position, but should not do this without assistance in case their oxygen levels drop during the turn. There are two ways the patient can position themselves in the prone position: either from a sitting or lying position.

Turning a conscious patient into the prone position

1. Explain the procedure to the patient and gain consent (Picture 9.1).
2. Prepare staff. All staff must be wearing personal protective equipment (PPE), FFP3 mask and goggles as per local and national guidelines. Assemble equipment: one to two pillows.

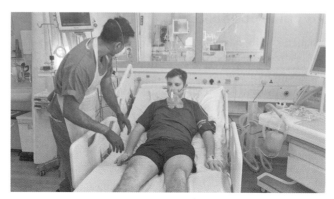

PICTURE 9.1   Explaining the procedure to the patient.

3. Assess the patient; consider increasing oxygen level (pre-oxygenation) prior to movement.
4. Check that the brakes on the bed are on and the bed rails are up. If turning from lying supine, both bed rails should be up, and for sitting position to prone, the furthest bed rail from the assistant should be raised.
5. Remove any non-essential infusions, for example, intravenous (IV) fluids for maintenance, electrocardiogram (ECG) electrodes and blood pressure cuff lead. Keep oxygen saturation probe attached, but check there is sufficient 'slack' in the cable (Picture 9.2).
6. Before laying the bed flat, if appropriate, increase oxygen, then lay the bed flat (Picture 9.3).

	Sitting to prone		**Lying supine**
7a.	Sit the patient on the edge of the bed, then lay the bed flat.	7b.	Ask the patient to move to one side of the bed, then lay the bed flat (Picture 9.4).
8a.	Ask the patient to lift their arms up above their head and turn to lie face down onto the bed (Picture 9.5).	8b.	Ask the patient to lift their arm above the head on the side that they will roll toward.
9a.	Ask/assist the patient to bring their legs onto the bed.	9b.	The patient then rolls themselves with or without assistance.

10. Advise the patient to put their head to one side (on a pillow) and check that CPAP/oxygen mask and tubing are not obstructed or kinked. If using a non-rebreath mask, check the bag is correctly inflated.
11. Arms can either be up at the head or in any comfortable position.
12. Check vital signs, including oxygen saturations, immediately.
13. Replace and check all monitoring equipment. Note that ECG electrodes should be placed on the patient's back. Any infusions should be restarted (Picture 9.6).

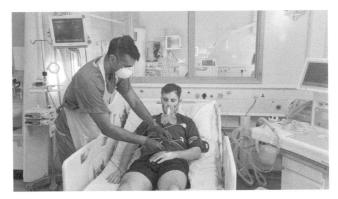

PICTURE 9.2   Remove all non-essential monitoring and infusions.

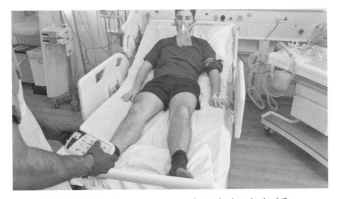

PICTURE 9.3   Increase oxygen prior to laying the bed flat.

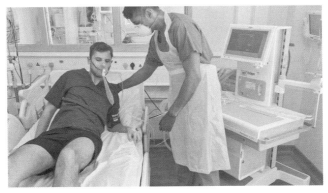

PICTURE 9.4   Ask/assist the patient to move to the side of the bed.

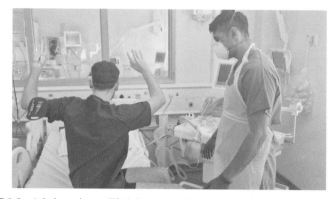

PICTURE 9.5   Ask the patient to lift their arms up above their head and turn to lie face down on the bed.

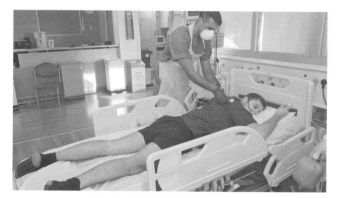

PICTURE 9.6   Replace and check all monitoring equipment.

14. The bed should be placed into the reverse Trendelenburg position (10–20 degrees) and vital signs rechecked in case of hypotension (Picture 9.7).
15. Check that the patient's call bell is within easy reach.
16. Maintain position for as long as possible.

De-proning

1. Complete steps 1–5 as outlined previously.
2. Reverse the procedure until the patient is either sitting upright, side lying or supine (steps 6–9).
3. Reassess the patient and complete steps 10–15.

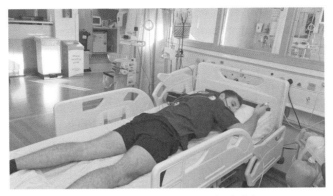

PICTURE 9.7   Recheck the patient's vital signs.

Prone position (unconscious)

During the pandemic, the increasing numbers of patients requiring prone positioning has led to the establishment of 'proning teams'. Led by an anaesthetist (or suitably trained advanced airway provider), the team is pretrained and when necessary is able to turn a patient into the prone or supine position. Local and national guidelines and checklists are being developed to guide and support these teams [4].

Careful monitoring of patients is essential as there is some evidence that the prone position has been associated with a higher incidence of adverse effects than identified in patients placed in the supine position [37]. Potential complications include airway obstruction from a kinked or displaced endotracheal tube (ETT). Once in the prone position, frequent oral suctioning and mouth care are required as secretions may reduce the integrity of ETT securing devices. In addition, proning can lead to facial swelling, causing retinal nerve compression, ETT ties can become too tight and pressure ulcers can develop. Electrodes for cardiac monitoring need to be applied posteriorly on the patient's back and in the event of cardiac arrest the anterior/posterior placement of defibrillator pads/paddles should be used [38]. Enteral feeding can continue in the prone position; however, the procedure is high risk for vomiting and/or increased gastric residual vomiting [39–41]. Absolute contraindications for prone position include spinal instability, unstable fractures, burns, open wounds, pregnancy, recent tracheal surgery and raised intracranial pressure. Relative contraindications include haemodynamic instability (including the use of vasopressors), cardiac pacemakers and abdominal surgery [37].

Neuromuscular blocking agents may be required to maintain gaseous exchange; this reduces extrapulmonary resistance and ventilatory desynchrony, which in turn results in improved oxygenation. Paralysis of the diaphragm allows for metabolic rest, reduced oxygen consumption and invasive control of breathing mechanics [26]. Neuromuscular blockage may be required in patients with ARDS as this allows for less PEEP to maintain oxygenation and reduced mortality.

Turning a patient into the prone position

1. Preparation (staff). All staff must be wearing PPE, FFP3 mask and goggles as per local and national guidelines. A minimum of five practitioners, including an airway-trained practitioner, are needed. During the preparation phase, the team members should introduce themselves and state their role. The airway-trained person should be positioned at the head end and is responsible for coordinating the procedure. At least two other people standing on either side of the patient will be needed; additional staff may be required to manage chest drains/ECMO cannulas, etc. and to make sure that correct positioning is maintained throughout the procedure. Equipment needed is listed in Table 9.2.

2. Preparation (patient). Enteral feeding must stop a minimum of 1 h prior to position change and the nasogastric tube aspirated and clamped, stopping any non-essential infusions, for example, maintenance of crystalloid infusions. Consideration should be given to temporarily removing monitoring equipment to prevent entanglement during moving. Where this is necessary, a full set of vital signs should be recorded immediately prior to starting the intervention. The airway-trained person (leader) must be able to see the monitor at all times.

3. Positioning. The patient should be laid flat in a neutral position and on a clean sheet with a slide sheet placed underneath. The arm closest to the ventilator is tucked underneath the buttock with the palm facing anteriorly. At this point the anterior ECG electrodes are removed. Pillows, if required, can be placed over the chest, iliac crests and knees. They should be placed strategically to reduce the pressure placed upon key areas.

TABLE 9.2 Equipment needed for prone positioning.

- Pressure-relieving mattress
- Airway trolley
- Closed-circuit suctioning
- Endotracheal tube tapes
- Eye ointment
- Slide sheet
- ×2 clean bedsheets
- ×3–5 pillows
- Electrocardiogram electrodes
- Absorbent pad

4. A clean bed sheet should be placed on top of the patient leaving only the head and neck exposed. The edges from the top and bottom bed sheets are rolled tightly together, encasing the patient between the two and keeping the pillows in the correct position on top of the patient (see Picture 9.8).

5. Stage 1: Keeping the bed sheets pulled taught and the edges rolled tight; the patient should be moved horizontally to lie on the edge of the bed (the direction should be away from the ventilator in the opposite direction to which the patient will be turned). On command from the leader, while maintaining a tight grip on the rolled-up sheets, the patient is rotated 90 degrees to lie on their side. Staff on either side should then adjust their hand positions on the rolled-up sheets so that they now have hold of the opposite edge when compared to the horizontal move (see Pictures 9.9–9.11).

6. Stage 2: On command, the rolled-up sheet is pulled up from beneath the patient while the patient is carefully turned into the prone position. With the airway person carefully supporting the head and neck, the head is turned to face the ventilator as the patient is moved from the lateral to the prone position (see Picture 9.12).

7. Stage 3: The endotracheal tube must be checked for kinks, correct positioning and that an $EtCO_2$ trace is still present. The ventilator settings should then be reviewed. ECG electrodes are then re-attached to the patient's back and all monitoring, infusions and enteral feed are re-established.

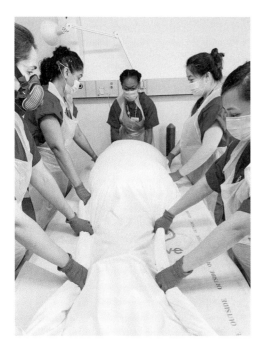

PICTURE 9.8 Positioning of staff for prone positioning.

PICTURE 9.9 Moving the patient horizontally away from the ventilator.

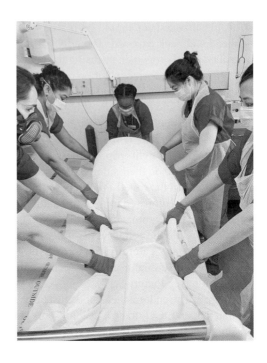

PICTURE 9.10 Rotating the patient to 90 degrees.

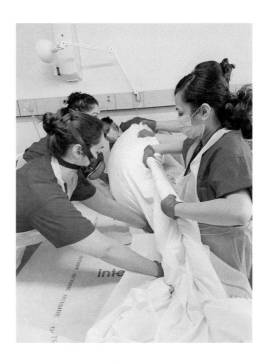

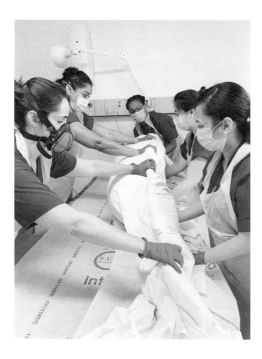

PICTURE 9.11   Hand position changes of staff.

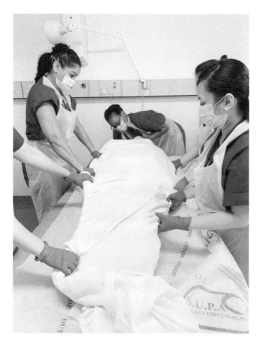

PICTURE 9.12   Patient in prone position.

TABLE 9.3 Nursing considerations for the prone position.

Indications	Potential complications
Moderate to severe acute respiratory distress syndrome with PaO_2:FiO_2 ratio <150 mmHg and FiO_2 ≥0.6 • Early use (ideally <48 h) following 12–24 h of mechanical ventilation • Lung-protective strategies • Use of neuromuscular blocking drugs if there is evidence of ventilator dysynchrony	• Pressure sores (most cited injury) • Facial/periorbital oedema • Intravenous line/endotracheal tube (ETT) displacement • Cardiovascular system instability • Ocular injury/corneal abrasions • Brachial plexus injury • Staff injury • Continuous renal replacement therapy line flow problems

Nursing considerations:

Check head is turned sufficiently to avoid kinking ETT and ventilator tubing

Electrocardiogram electrodes removed from front and placed on back (reversed) as indicated using colour coding

Nurse on pressure-relieving mattress

Bed head elevation >25 degrees

Change head and arm positions (swimmer's position) every 2–4 h

Consider neuromuscular blockade. Deep sedation (Richmond Agitation and Sedation Score –5)

Check pressure areas:

• Direct pressure on the eyes

• Ears not bent over

• ETT not pressed against the corner of the mouth/lips

• Nasogastric tube is not pressed against the nostril

• Male patient's penis is between the legs

• Urinary catheter secured

• Any lines and tubing not pressed against the skin

8. Stage 4: If necessary, the patient should be moved into the centre of the bed, the slide sheet removed and an absorbent pad placed under the patient's head to catch any oral secretions. The patient's arms should be carefully positioned in the 'swimmer's position' by raising one arm on the same side as the head is facing, while placing the other arm by the patient's side. The shoulder should be abducted to 80 degrees and the elbow flexed 90 degrees on the raised arm. In addition, the spine and limbs need to be kept in neutral alignment. The patient should be nursed at 30 degrees in the reverse Trendelenburg position (Table 9.3).

9. Pressure area care. Check all pillow positions to confirm optimal positioning. Pressure areas should be carefully and fully checked so that there is no direct pressure on the eyes, the ears are not bent over, the ETT is not pressed against the corner of the mouth/lips, the nasogastric tube is not pressed against the nostril, the penis is hanging between the legs with the catheter secured and any lines and tubing are not pressed against the skin.

Once turned into the prone position, patients may remain in this position for 12–16 h per day [42]. In addition, patients may need to be placed into this position several times. Patients in the prone position should be nursed on a pressure-relieving mattress to reduce pressure damage and it will be necessary to change the position of the head and arms every 2–4 h. To maintain the prone position, ventilated patients must be adequately sedated with the use of neuromuscular blockade [37,43].

It is important to note that critically ill patients are at high risk of developing malnutrition and sarcopenia [44]. Therefore it is accepted practice that early enteral feeding should be established unless contraindicated; in addition, the enteral route is preferred over the parenteral route (e.g., total parenteral nutrition [39, 40], [41]). However, there is an increased risk of gastric aspiration during repositioning; therefore interruptions in the enteral feeding regimens have to occur when positioning a patient from supine to prone and vice versa. Enteral feeding should be resumed once the patient has been repositioned, nasogastric tube position confirmed and vital signs recorded.

Research into the impact of the prone position on tolerance and gastrointestinal complications is still ongoing. De la Fuente et al.'s [40] small-scale study of enteral feeding tolerance in ventilated prone patients concluded that enteral feeding did not increase the risk of gastrointestinal problems. In contrast, Malhotra et al. [37] found that patients in the prone position developed a higher incidence of vomiting and/or an increase in gastric residual volumes. As a result of their findings, Malhotra et al. [37] recommend patients' heads should be elevated at least 25 degrees while receiving enteral feeding and that prokinetic drugs such as erythromycin may be appropriate.

Conclusion

Nurses need understanding of the complex pathophysiological processes that arise from COVID-19 infection. However, as this chapter has indicated, the pathophysiology associated with the development of COVID-19-related ARDS is still being investigated. Nevertheless, the high incidence of ARDS in COVID-19 patients has resulted in the recognition that use of the prone position undertaken early for both conscious and unconscious patients can improve oxygenation. It has been identified as an intervention that for some patients may reduce or avoid the need for invasive ventilation. Nevertheless, it has to be accepted that it poses potential risks and complications. Protocols, guidelines and training are essential to minimize the risk of adverse events during or after prone positioning. The COVID-19 pandemic is relatively new; therefore further research is needed before definitive guidelines and recommendations can be made.

References

[1] Ghelichkhani P, Esmaeili M. Prone position in management of COVID-19 patients; a commentary. Arch Acad Emergency Med 2020;8(1):e48.

[2] Seaton-Mills D. Prone positioning in ARDS: a nursing perspective. Clin Intensive Care 2000;11(4):203–8.

[3] Telias I, Katira BH, Brochard L. Is the prone position helpful during spontaneous breathing in patients with COVID-19. J Am Med Assoc 2020;323(22):2265–7.

[4] Intensive Care Society. Guidance for: prone positioning in adult critical care. 2019. www.ics. ac.uk.

[5] Centre for Disease Control and Prevention. Interim considerations for infection prevention and control of coronavirus diseases 2019 (COVID-19) in obstetric healthcare settings. 2020. https://www.cdc.gov/coronavirus/2019-ncov/hcp/disposition-hospitalized-patients.html.

[6] Yang D, Leibowitz JL. The structure and functions of coronavirus genomic 3′ and 5′ ends. Virus Res 2015;206:120–33. https://doi.org/10.1016/j.virusres.2015.02.025.

[7] Chad T, Sampson C. Prone positioning in conscious patients on medical wards: a review of the evidence and its relevance to patients with COVID-19 infection. Clin Med 2020;20(4):e97–103.

[8] Marini JJ, Gattinoni L. Management of COVID-19 respiratory distress. J Am Med Assoc 2020;323(22):2329–30.

[9] Dhont S, et al. The pathophysiology of 'happy' hypoxemia in Covid-19. Respir Res 2020;21:198.

[10] Tobin MJ, Laghi F, Jubran A. Why COVID-19 silent hypoxemia is baffling to physicians. Am J Respir Crit Care Med 2020;202(3):356–60. https://doi.org/10.1164/rccm.202006-2157CP. PMID: 32539537; PMCID: PMC7397783.

[11] Xie J, Covassin N, Fan Z, Singh P, Gao W, Li G, Kara T, Somers VK, et al. Association between hypoxemia and mortality in patients with COVID-19. Mayo Clin Proc 2020;95(6):1138–47.

[12] Jain A, Doyle DJ. Stages or phenotypes? A critical look at COVID-19 pathophysiology. Intensive Care Med 2020;46(7):1494–5.

[13] Coperchinia F, Chiovato L, Crocea L, Magria F, Rotondi M. The cytokine storm in COVID-19: an overview of the involvement of the chemokine/chemokine-receptor system. Cytokine Growth Factor Rev 2020;53:25–32.

[14] Wilcox S. Management of respiratory failure due to covid-19. BMJ 2020;329:m1786.

[15] Mohlenkamp S, Thiele H. Ventilation of COVID-19 patients in intensive care units. Herz 2020;45(4):329–31. https://doi.org/10.1007/s00059-020-04923-1.

[16] Ashbaugh DG, Bigelow DB, Petty TL, Levine BE. Acute respiratory distress in adults. Lancet 1967;12(2):319–23. 7511.

[17] Bernard GR, Artigas A, Brigham KL, Carlet J, Falke K, Hudson L, Lamy M, Legall JO, Morris A, Spragg R. The American-European Consensus Conference on ARDS. Definitions, mechanisms, relevant outcomes and clinical trial co-ordination. Am J Respir Crit Care Med 1994;149(3 Pt 1):818–24.

[18] Ferguson ND, Fan E, Camporota L, Antonelli M, Anzueto A, Beale R, Brochard L, Brower R, Esteban A, Gattinoni L, Rhodes A, Slutsky AS, Vincent JL, Rubenfeld GD, Thompson BT, Tanieri VM. The Berlin Definition of ARDS: an expanded rationale, justification and supplementary material. Intensive Care Med 2012;38(10):1573–82.

[19] Ranieri VM, Rubenfeld G, Thompson BT. Acute respiratory distress syndrome: the Berlin definition. J Am Med Assoc 2012;307(23):2526–33.

[20] Fanelli V, Vlachou A, Ghannadian S, Simonetti U, Slutsky AS, Zhang H. Acute respiratory distress syndrome: new definition, current and future therapeutic options. J Thorac Dis 2013;5(3):326–34. https://doi.org/10.3978/j.issn.2072-1439.2013.04.05.

[21] ARDS Definition Task Force. Acute respiratory distress syndrome: the Berlin definition. J Am Med Assoc 2012;307:2526–33.

[22] Villar J, Perez-Mendez L, Blanco J, Anon JM, Blanch L, Belda J, Santos-Bouza A, Fenandez RL, Kacmarek RM. Spanish initiative for epidemiology, stratification, and therapies for

ARDS (SIESTA) network. A universal definition of ARDS: the PaO_2/FiO_2 ratio under a standard ventilator setting- a prospective, multicentre validation study. Intensive Care Med 2013;39:583–92.

[23] Pelosi P, D'Onofrio D, Chiumello D, Paolo S, Chiara G, Capelozzi VL, Barbas CS, Chiaranda M, Gattinoni L. Pulmonary and extra pulmonary acute respiratory distress syndrome are different. Eur Respir J 2003;22:48s–56s.

[24] Tremblay L, Valenza F, Ribeiro SP, Slutsky AS. Injurious ventilator strategies increase cytokines and c-fos m-RNA expression in an isolated rat lung model. J Clin Invest 1997;99(5):944–52.

[25] European Society of Intensive Care Medicine. Acute respiratory distress syndrome. 2nd ed. 2017. www.esicm.org.

[26] Baid H. Patient safety: identifying and managing complications of mechanical ventilation. Crit Care Nurs Clin N Am 2016;28:451–62.

[27] Pooni RS. Research in brief: prone positioning in COVID-19: what's the evidence?. Royal College of Physicians London; 2020.

[28] Bamford P, Bentley A, Dean J, Whitmore D, Wilson-Baig N. ICS guidance for prone positioning of the conscious COVID patient 2020. 2020. www.ics.ac.org.

[29] Rimmer A, Wilkinson E. What's happening in covid-19 ICUs? An intensive care doctor answers some common questions. BMJ 2020;369:m1552.

[30] Riviello ED, Kiviri W, Twagirumugabe T, Mueller A, Banner-Goodspeed VM, Officer L, Novack V, Mutumwinka M, Talmor DS, Fowler RA. Hospital incidence and outcomes of the acute respiratory distress syndrome using the Kigali modification of the Berlin definition. Am J Respir Crit Care Med 2020;193(1):52–9. https://doi.org/10.1164/rccm.201503-0584OC.

[31] Bryan AC. Comments of a devil's advocate. Am Rev Respir Dis 1974;110(Suppl. l):143–4.

[32] Geurin C, Gaillard S, Lemasson S. Effects of systematic prone positioning in hypoxaemic acute respiratory failure. J Am Med Assoc 2004;292:2379–87.

[33] Mancebo J, Fernández R, Blanch L, et al. A multicenter trial of prolonged prone ventilation in severe acute respiratory distress syndrome. Am J Respir Crit Care Med 2006;173:1233–9.

[34] Taccone P, Pesenti A, Latini R, Prone–Supine II Study Group, et al. Prone positioning in patients with moderate and severe acute respiratory distress syndrome: a randomized controlled trial. J Am Med Assoc 2009;302:1977–84.

[35] Gattinoni L, Tognoni G, Pesenti A, et al. Effect of prone positioning on the survival of patients with acute respiratory failure. N Engl J Med 2001;345(8):568–73.

[36] Sud S, Friedrich J, Adhikari N, et al. Effect of prone positioning during mechanical ventilation on mortality among patients with acute respiratory distress syndrome: a systematic review and meta-analysis. CMAJ 2014;186(10):381–90.

[37] Malhotra A, Kacmarek RM, Parsons PE, Finlay G. Prone ventilation for adults patients with acute respiratory distress syndrome. 2020. https://www.uptodate.com/contents/prone-ventilation-for-adult-patients-with-acute-respiratory-distress-syndrome#H2655777180.

[38] Poston JT, Patel BK, Davis AM. Management of critically ill adults with COVID-19. J Am Med Assoc 2020;323(18):1839–41. https://doi.org/10.1001/jama.2020.4914.

[39] Riegner J, Thenoz-Jist N, Fiancette M, et al. Early enteral nutrition in mechanically ventilated patients in the prone position. Crit Care Med 2004;32:94.

[40] De la Fuente I, De la Fuente J, Estelles M, et al. Enteral Nutrition in Patients Receiving Mechanical Ventilation in a Prone Position. JPEN J Parenter Enteral Nutr 2016;40(2):250–5. https://doi.org/10.1177/0148607114553232.

[41] Hardy G, Bharal M, Clemente R, Hammond R, Wandrag L. BDA Critical Care Specialist Group COVID-19 Best Practice Guidance: Enteral Feeding in Prone Position. 2020. Version 1.0 - 08/04/2020.

[42] Beeching N, Fletcher T, Fowler R. Coronavirus disease 2019. HYPERLINK. 2020. http://www.bestpractice.bmj.com. www.bestpractice.bmj.com.

[43] Garrett KM. Best practices for managing pain, sedation and delirium in the mechanically ventilated patient. Crit Care Nurse Clin N Am 2016;28:437–50.

[44] Thibault R, Seguin P, Tamion F, et al. Nutrition of the COVID-19 patient in the intensive care unit (ICU): a practical guidance. Crit Car 2020;24:447. https://doi.org/10.1186/s13054-020-03159-z.

Chapter 10

Haemodynamic assessment, monitoring and management

Chris Carter, Joy Notter

Chapter Outline

In severe COVID-19, a key characteristic of the disease is respiratory failure, often without accompanying circulatory failure. While it is accepted that although haemodynamic instability is not common in COVID-19 patients, nurses must include cardiovascular assessment as part of comprehensive patient appraisal [1]. Haemodynamic instability may occur because of fever, fluid restrictions to prevent pulmonary oedema in patients with severe acute respiratory distress syndrome (ARDS) or sepsis due to complications of COVID-19 or nosocomial infection [1]. In this chapter, haemodynamic considerations when managing a patient with severe COVID-19 disease will be considered. Both critical care and redeployed nurses working as key frontline staff in response to the pandemic must be competent in basic and advanced haemodynamic monitoring, as they need to recognize, interpret and respond to evolving patient status.

Patient assessment

As outlined in Chapter 6, haemodynamic assessment provides an overview of key aspects of cardiovascular assessment. In critical care, patients may be continuously monitored [2], but this does not negate the need for completion of a holistic physical assessment of the patient, which includes both basic and advanced cardiac assessment.

The COVID-19 pandemic has impacted on all processes in critical care, limiting the availability of resources that in high-income countries have traditionally been taken for granted. However, an international survey during the COVID-19 pandemic confirmed that almost all critical care units continued to use central venous catheters for drug administration, central venous pressure (CVP) monitoring and mixed venous oxygen saturations. Invasive blood pressure (BP) was predominantly measured using a radial arterial line, with a few units reporting the use of femoral lines (157/998 = 16%) and the oscillometric brachial cuff method (173/998%=17%) [1].

Electrocardiogram

Electrocardiogram (ECG) monitoring identifies heart rate, rhythm and the presence of ischaemia or infarction, electrolyte imbalance or other abnormalities, detecting changes in condition and responses to therapy in real time [2]. Cardiac monitors have alarms, which need to be set to identify any significant changes in condition, and settings must be checked for safe physiological limits for each patient [3]. Continuous cardiac monitoring with three of five leads is the most commonly used method for monitoring heart rate and rhythm. ECG cables are usually colour coded; the UK colours are given next. In some countries such as the United States, colour codes may vary [4]. They should be placed:

1. Red electrode to the right shoulder.
2. Yellow electrode to the left shoulder.
3. Green electrode to the left side of the upper abdominal wall.

Lead 2 offers the best view and should be used as the default setting for monitoring [4]. In addition to noting the cardiac rhythm, it is good practice to palpate a patient's pulse even if it is shown on a pulse oximeter, automatic BP machine or cardiac monitor so that the strength and rhythm of the pulse are documented, in addition to the rate. Palpation should register the rate, rhythm, pressure (volume) and if appropriate deficits with the apex beat [3].

Interpreting cardiac rhythms

A typical adult heart rate is between 60 and 100 beats per minute. A rate of less than 60 beats per minute is termed bradycardia and a rate of over 100 beats per minute is termed tachycardia. In sinus rhythm, as the atria depolarize, a P wave is seen on the monitor, followed by ventricular contraction (QRS wave) and finally repolarization (T wave) [4,5] (Fig. 10.1).

If the heart rate changes, or if there is a change in BP or a change in conscious level (which may trigger an alarm), the nurse must immediately respond and assess the patient, and where appropriate call for help (Fig. 10.2).

Sinus rhythm

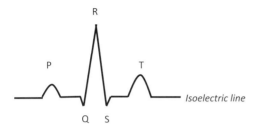

Bradycardia rate <60 beats per minute
Tachycardia rate >100 beats per minute

FIGURE 10.1   Sinus rhythm.

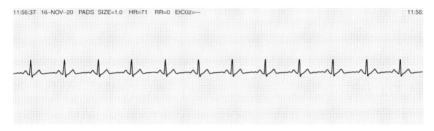

FIGURE 10.2   Sinus rhythm waveform.

To interpret a cardiac rhythm, a printed rhythm strip is needed. Although there are several ways to interpret cardiac rhythms, a practical example of a commonly used method is illustrated next [4].

- Step 1: Is there any electrical activity and a pulse? If there is no pulse, check that a lead has not become disconnected and reassess the patient; if there is still no pulse, immediately begin cardiopulmonary resuscitation (Chapter 13).
- Step 2: Work out the ventricular (QRS) rate. ECG paper is calibrated in mm, with bolder lines every 5 mm. Standard ECG paper speed is 25 mm^{-3}. Therefore every five large squares or 25 small squares equals 1 s. To work out the rate, count the number of cardiac cycles (R-to-R wave) that occurs in 6 s (30 large squares) and multiply by 10. This provides an estimated heart rate, even when the beat is irregular. For shorter rhythm strips, count the number of cardiac cycles in 3 s (15 large squares) and multiply by 20.
- Step 3: Assess if the QRS rhythm is regular or irregular. This may be obvious; however, if unsure, take a piece of paper, mark several R waves on the paper and then move the paper along to see if it matches up with other R waves. If the dots/marks line up, the rhythm is regular; if they do not, then it is irregular.
- Step 4: Check the QRS complex duration. The normal duration is <0.12 s or three small squares. This will identify a broad or narrow arrhythmia, for example, pulsed ventricular tachycardia (broad) or atrial flutter (narrow).

TABLE 10.1 Common cardiac arrhythmias [4,6].

Type	Description
Sinus Bradycardia	Sinus bradycardia is a heart rate less than 60 beats per minute. Bradycardia may be a physiological state of very fit people, or during sleep, or as a result of beta-blocker therapy. Pathological bradycardia may be caused by a problem with the sinoatrial node or from complete failure of the atrioventricular conduction
Sinus Tachycardia	A heart rate of greater than 100 beats per minute
Atrial Fibrillation (AF)	AF is a common arrhythmia seen in clinical practice. It is characterized by disorganized electrical activity in the atria, no recognizable P waves, or coordinated atrial activity. The rate can be between 160 and 180 beats per minute. Common causes: hypertension, obesity, excessive alcohol intake or heart disease

- Step 5: Check if atrial (P wave) activity is present. It may be difficult to assess this as other factors may partially or fully occlude the trace, for example, tachycardia. If this is the case, the lack of a clear P wave should be recorded.
- Step 6: Assess whether the atrial (P wave) activity is related to ventricular (QRS complex) activity, and if so, how? If there is no relationship between the P and QRS waves, this indicates dissociation between the atrial and ventricular mechanisms of conduction. Examples may include heart blocks.

Common arrhythmias in critical care include sinus bradycardia, sinus tachycardia, atrial fibrillation and supraventricular tachycardia (Table 10.1). It is important to note that, in COVID-19, potential causes of arrhythmias may be due to viral myocardial damage, hypoxia, hypotension, heightened inflammatory status, reduced ACE-2 receptor activation and drug toxicity [7]. Although current data suggests the use of hydroxychloroquine or chloroquine does not reduce deaths among hospitalized patients with COVID-19, it may be appropriate in moderate disease; however, further research is required [8]. If these drugs are used, they may have a cardiac effect, for example, increased depolarization length causing an arrhythmia, and hydroxychloroquine is known to cause QT prolongation [7]. In consequence, understanding cardiac monitoring is a crucial aspect of patient care.

If an abnormality is detected, a 12-lead ECG should be performed and investigated further as part of an overall assessment for adverse signs (e.g., chest pain, cardiac failure, syncope, etc.), fluid loss and electrolyte imbalances [2].

Heart sounds

The wearing of personal protective equipment (PPE) may prevent the use of stethoscopes, as this may breach the integrity of the PPE. However, where possible, the nurse should palpate for the apex beat. The aortic, pulmonary, tricuspid and mitral valve areas should be auscultated, as should any additional sounds such as clicks and heart murmurs. The normal heart sounds are S1 (lub) and S2 (dub), while additional sounds, such as blowing, whooshing or rasping, may be indicative of heart murmurs [9].

Transducing

In many critical care settings, invasive monitoring of BP and CVP is now deemed a universal aspect of monitoring in an unstable critically ill patient. Transducing is the process whereby an arterial line or central line provides a waveform and continuous reading. Lines are attached to a transducer-giving set, which amplifies the signal; this then undergoes an analogue-to-digital conversion and BP is displayed in real time. The system must be calibrated and zeroed for each patient at regular intervals and before each reading. This includes confirming the transducer remains in the correct position and poor traces (termed dampened signals) corrected to improve accuracy. The correct position for the transducer table is in line with the right atrium (mid-axillary line; phlebostatic axis). This anatomical reference point on the chest is used as the baseline for consistent transducer site placement. Invasive lines are kept patent by the transducer-giving set being attached to a bag of 0.9% normal saline and in a pressure bag inflated to 300 mmHg. This provides a continuous infusion of 3 mL/h to each line to maintain line patency. In addition, lines can be 'flushed' after blood sampling or drug administration via the central line.

Invasive blood pressure monitoring

Arterial BP can be continuously monitored on a beat-to-beat basis using an arterial cannula connected to a transducer-giving set. Arterial cannulation also allows for intermittent arterial blood gases and routine blood sampling. The most common site is the radial artery; however, brachial and femoral arteries may be used in hypovolaemic patients in extremis [2]. Indications for arterial BP include patients at risk of signs of deterioration, for example, haemodynamically unstable patients (blood loss or hypovolaemia), those requiring vasopressor infusions, and those who are post-operative [2,3].

Central venous pressure

Similar to invasive BP monitoring, CVP measurements can be continuously recorded using a transducer set. The tip of the CVP (also termed the central line, central venous catheter [CVC]), is usually sited in the superior vena cava or right atrium via the internal jugular or subclavian vein. CVP measures the volume of blood returning to the right atrium by measuring the pressure on the walls of the right atrium. Just as with arterial monitoring, the position of the transducer table can affect readings, and correct positioning needs to be checked prior to recording any observations.

CVP provides an estimate of the right ventricle end-diastolic pressure, which is an indication of right ventricular preload. However, it can be affected by positive-pressure ventilation and changes in ventricular and vascular tree compliance; therefore it can be an unreliable indicator in the assessment of intravascular fluid status or response to volume challenges.

Central venous oxygen saturation is an alternative (although not as accurate) for measuring mixed venous oxygen saturation (SvO_2) from a pulmonary artery catheter and indicates global oxygen supply and demand [2]. In the absence of a pulmonary artery catheter, central venous oxygen saturation provides a useful marker for the adequacy of global oxygen delivery and may be useful in targeted resuscitation. The normal SvO_2 is 60%–80%. A decrease in SvO_2 indicates oxygen transport and uptake may be inadequate due to increased cellular oxygen demand or decreased oxygen delivery. Alternatively, a high SvO_2 may be caused by high FiO_2 or reduced oxygen demand [3].

Neurovascular observations

In COVID-19 it is important to recognize that patients may have additional trauma or co-morbidities that must also be identified and treated [10]. Also, COVID-19 may affect coagulation and evidence is accruing that there may be microthrombi formation [11]. Therefore neurovascular observations, which assess for neurovascular compromise or acute compartment syndrome, are part of all critical care assessments.

Neurovascular perfusion should be assessed regularly using the 'five Ps' to assess perfusion: pain, pallor, paraesthesia, pulses and paralysis [10]. However, for patients in critical care, conventional methods of assessment used to assess neurovascular perfusion may be difficult due to communication limitations. In the event of signs of compartment syndrome to decrease tissue pressure, restore blood flow and reduce tissue damage and potential functional loss of the limb, an emergency fasciotomy is required. Wounds are then left open for at least 48 h until the pressure has reduced [10].

Central and peripheral capillary refill

Capillary refill time (CRT) is a simple bedside test to determine the measurement of hypovolaemia because of haemorrhage or dehydration [12]. Peripheral CRT is measured by holding the nailbed of a finger in line with the heart for 5 s; when released, the length of time the colour takes to return should be noted. When measuring central CRT, pressure should be applied to the patient's sternum or forehead and held for 5 s; the length of time for the colour to return should be noted. Normal capillary refill rate is under 2 s [13].

Skin integrity, colour and temperature

In COVID-19, patients may develop pyrexia and/or hypoxia; this assesses the patient's skin needs to include recognition of the range of potential causes of skin colour and temperature. For example, signs of pallor (pale, cold and clammy), anaemia by checking mucous membranes, for example, inside the lips or lower eyelids, jaundice, flushing, central or peripheral cyanosis and any scars.

Oedema

Oedema, is the collection of fluid in the tissue caused by abnormal fluid distribution and is not uncommon in critical care, but assessment needs to take account of any pre-existing co-morbidities and complications arising from the need for critical care [3]. To assess oedema, pressure is applied firmly over a bony prominence for 5 s, depending on the severity of oedema, it may result in retention of a finger imprint, termed 'pitting' oedema.

Temperature

Fever is a protective response for infections and an important criterion in the diagnosis of COVID-19 [14]. Initially, fever was reported in over 98% of patients [15–17]. However, there is increasing evidence that patients may be afebrile [18,19], while still infectious; therefore fever must not be used in isolation as a key indicator for COVID-19. The patient's core temperature should be measured using the oral route, the axilla or tympanic membrane. Other methods of temperature measurement the use of rectal thermometers or via invasive monitoring, for example, Swan Ganz catheter, PiCCO. However, the sublingual (oral) route is rarely used in critical care as patients tend to be intubated or may have tight-fitting masks due to CPAP or BiPAP.

Checking for signs of DVT

Critically ill patients are immobile and at increased risk of developing a deep vein thrombosis (DVT). In addition, while limited evidence is available regarding the incidence of DVT in critically ill COVID-19 patients, recent studies have identified that where there is a highly increased inflammatory response, there are increased rates of thrombotic events [11,19,20]. The calves should be assessed for signs of swelling and inflammation. The patient's drug chart should be checked to confirm if DVT prophylaxis has been prescribed and administered. Patients may wear antiembolism DVT stockings, and these should be monitored and taken down to assess for pressure damage on the heels and toes.

Advanced haemodynamic monitoring

In unstable critically ill patients, blood pressure is a poor marker of tissue and oxygen perfusion [2]. Therefore cardiac output (CO) monitoring may be more

TABLE 10.2 Factors affecting systemic vascular resistance (SVR) [3].

Low SVR	High SVR
Vasodilator therapy	Hypovolaemia
Sepsis	Hypothermia
Hyperdynamic septic shock	Cardiogenic shock
Cirrhosis	Vasopressors, e.g., noradrenaline
Aortic regurgitation	
Anaemia	
Anaphylactic and neurogenic shock	

appropriate to guide goal-directed cardiovascular support therapies, for example, vasopressor or vasoactive drugs. CO is the amount of blood ejected from the left ventricle into the aorta per minute. It is dependent on the amount of blood ejected each heart beat (stroke volume) multiplied by the heart rate in a minute. Normal CO is 4–8 L/min. A more accurate assessment is to use the cardiac index (CI), which provides CO based on the patient's body size. To calculate the CI, CO is divided by the patient's body surface area (height and weight). Normal CI in adults ranges from 2.5 to 4.2 L/min/m².

Stroke volume is the amount of blood ejected by the ventricle during each contraction (systole), which is approximately 70 mL. Some CO monitors allow continuous CO monitoring and the value is updated every 30–60 s [22]. Using this technique allows for real-time detection of complications and monitoring of the patient's condition.

Systemic vascular resistance (SVR) is the resistance to blood flow in the entire systemic circulation. SVR ranges from 9.6 to 18.8 min/L (770–1500 dyn/s/cm⁵). Factors affecting SVR are outlined in Table 10.2. SVR is calculated by:

$$SRV = (MAP - CVP)/80 \times CO\,(L/m)$$

CO monitoring includes invasive and non-invasive methods. The pulmonary artery catheter (PAC) was developed in the 1970s and was deemed the gold standard method for CO measurement, until the advent of a large international randomized-control trial on the use of PAC versus other methods of CO monitoring. The study concluded there was no clear evidence of benefit or harm in using a PAC [21]. In consequence, the study exposed units to different methods of CO monitoring and resulted in many critical care units adopting less invasive methods. In consequence, a variety of CO methods are now used in practice. Methods of invasive CO monitoring include pulmonary artery catheter, dilution techniques and arterial pulse contour analysis (e.g., LiDCO, Pulsion medical system, PiCCO) and non-invasive methods include oesophageal Doppler and echocardiography methods (Table 10.3). An international review of critical care practices during COVID-19 by Michard et al. [1] identified that haemodynamic instability was not uncommon in critically ill patients. Monitoring included

TABLE 10.3 Invasive and non-invasive methods of cardiac output monitoring [2,3,22].

Invasive methods	Pulmonary artery catheter	The pulmonary artery catheter is a long catheter generally inserted through the internal jugular and the distal port of the catheter with a balloon on the end that sits in the pulmonary artery. The balloon 'floats' the catheter in the direction of blood flow until the tip reaches the branch of the pulmonary artery. The catheter has a lumen to inflate/deflate the balloon and a proximal lumen in the right atrium to measure central venous pressure (CVP). When the balloon is deflated, the pulmonary artery pressure is shown and indirectly measures the left ventricle's end-diastolic pressure (LVEDP) and is useful when managing an unstable haemodynamically compromised patient. The average systolic pressure is 20–30 mmHg and diastolic pressure is between 8 and 15 mmHg. When the balloon is inflated (termed 'wedged'), the right pressure becomes blocked for a short period and the pulmonary artery wedge pressure (PAWP) is measured and reflects the left atrial pressure, LVEDP and the left ventricle preload. The PAWP is deemed more reliable than CVP and is generally between 5 and 12 mmHg. Other lumens of the pulmonary artery catheter can be used for infusions and medications. There is also a thermistor that measures the core body temperature
	Arterial pulse contour analysis	This uses either boluses of cold injector or a thermal filament within the catheter emitting a pulse of heat. As the temperature change is detected by a thermistor located at the tip of the catheter, this generates a curve, which is proportional to cardiac output (CO). Lithium can also be used instead of cold boluses of fluid, which is then detected via a lithium-sensitive electrode in blood sampled from an arterial cannula
Non-invasive methods	Echocardiography	Systemic arterial pressure waveforms are analysed on a beat-to-beat basis to estimate CO
	Transoesophageal echocardiography	This is an ultrasound probe placed into the oesophagus via the mouth or nose. By measuring the velocity of blood flow in the descending aorta, the velocity of descending blood flow is measured by the Doppler effect. During diastole blood flow is not moving, the wave is the same frequency as the emitted wave. Whereas, during systole blood is moving away from the probe, the wave changes. The faster the blood flow, the greater the drop in frequency. CO is measured by assessing size, shape and changes in the shape of velocity waveforms in the descending aorta, demonstrating increasing resistance. Waveform shapes can provide information on ventricular preload, afterload and contractility

TABLE 10.4 Common types of vasopressors and inotropes used in critical care [2,23].

Drug	Dose range	Receptor	Effects
Noradrenaline (norepinephrine)	0.01–1 mcg/kg/min	α	↑SVR
Adrenaline (epinephrine)	1 mg intravenous in cardiac arrest	β1 β2 α	↑Contractility ↑SVR ↑HR
Dobutamine	2.5–20 mcg/kg/min	β1++ β2+	↑Contractility ↓SVR ↑HR
Dopexamine	0.5–6 mcg/kg/min	β1 β2	↑Contractility ↓SVR ↑HR
Dopamine	1–5 mcg/kg/min 5–10 mcg/kg/min >10 mcg/kg/min	DA1 β1 α	↓Renal SVR ↑Contractility ↑HR ↑SVR

HR, heart rate; *SVR*, systemic vascular resistance.

central venous oxygen saturation measurement from the CVC (94%) and ultrasounds were the most common method used to predict fluid responsiveness and assess pulmonary oedema and cardiac function.

Pump up the pressure: fluid versus vasopressors

The initial priority in a patient with poor perfusion is to maintain reasonable haemodynamic status while the cause of shock and its pathogenesis are identified and addressed. Haemodynamic therapy can be categorized into fluid resuscitation, vasopressor therapy and inotropic therapy.

Not all patients with cardiovascular instability will need treatment with vasoactive drugs. Initially, correction of fluid balance may improve cardiovascular parameters, increasing perfusion and oxygen delivery and reducing the need for vasopressors [3]. However, patients with profound haemodynamic impairment will need vasoactive or inotrope therapy to restore tissue perfusion in shock states. Vasopressors increase BP by causing arteriole vasoconstriction. Inotropes increase myocardial contractility [3,23]. Table 10.4 outlines commonly used vasopressors and inotropes. Vasopressors and inotropes work on α, β1, β2 and DA1 receptor sites [23].

- α receptor sites are located in the coronary arterioles and vascular smooth muscle; they increase SVR and in turn increase BP.

TABLE 10.5 Nursing considerations.

Close monitoring:
- Continuous electrocardiogram (ECG), arterial blood pressure, SpO_2, +/– advanced haemodynamic monitoring
- Accurate fluid balance – input and output
- Monitor blood sugar levels
- Monitor pressure areas, peripheries for blanching/cyanosis, for signs of extravasation
- Correct prescription/dose:
  - Check sufficient supply of prepared drug
  - Check accurate drug calculations
  - Check correct documentation
- Equipment is functioning properly and plugged in continuous power supply
- 'Double pumping' (see later)
- Record 12-lead ECG daily
- Use a dedicated line for administration of vasopressor infusions
- All syringes containing drugs should be labelled with the appropriate drug label in a place where it can be clearly seen and include the date and time
- Depending on local policy and protocols, lines will be labelled at the syringe pump and patient end and will include the date and time the line was first used; this will indicate when the line should be changed (Fig. 10.3)

- β1 receptors are located in the sinoatrial node and myocardium; when stimulated they increase heart rate and myocardial contractility.
- β2 receptor sites are located in the coronary arterioles, bronchial smooth muscle, atrioventricular node and vascular smooth muscle; when stimulated they cause an increase in contractility and a reduction in SVR.
- DA1 are found in the kidneys and myocardium; when stimulated they cause vasodilation.

Vasopressor therapy

The use of vasopressor and positive inotropes in critical care is a common aspect of patient care [23]. Staff redeployed into critical care should not be expected to care for patients requiring vasopressors unsupervised, unless they have been trained and formally assessed as competent (Table 10.5).

Vasopressors are not curative; they are designed to support the patient's condition while definitive therapy is established. Thus an infusion may be commenced to support a patient with a compromised haemodynamic status, for example, due to septic shock, and hypotension caused by sedation-related side effects [23,24]. Potential complications of initiating vasopressor infusions can be systemic and may include increased myocardial oxygen consumption, gut and limb ischaemia, hyperglycaemia, changes in the immune response to infection and pressure ulcers [23–25]. In addition, vasopressor drugs can have an effect on myocardial contractility and SVR by either causing vasoconstriction or vasodilation. Dosage is

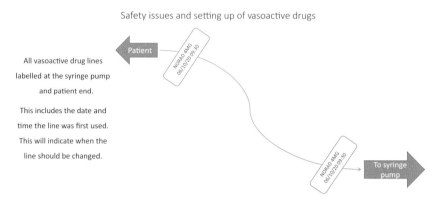

FIGURE 10.3   Syringe pump diagram for setting up vasoactive drugs.

calculated in micrograms per kilogram per minute (mcg/kg/min). They are usually administered via central access and titrated to achieve individual specific targets, for example, mean arterial pressure (MAP) >65 mmHg.

Vasopressors are high-risk drugs due to their rapid effect on the cardiovascular system and their short duration of action. Continuous infusions of these drugs are necessary to maintain a constant plasma drug concentration; they *must not* be stopped and any alarms dealt with immediately. A replacement syringe should be prepared well in advance of the old syringe needing to be replaced. Note that there can be serious consequences if the drug administration routes are not rigorously monitored.

Double pumping

Double pumping is terminology for a situation whereby one vasopressor infusion is substituted for another without interrupting the flow of the drug to a patient, for a seamless transition between one infusion ending and another commencing. This maintains cardiovascular stability by providing a continuous flow of the infusion and prevention of the discontinuation of therapy. It is important to note that each critical care team will have its own specific protocol for double pumping of vasopressors. The patient should never be left unattended during the double-pumping procedure. In patients who become hypotensive during the syringe change, or whose BP is unresponsive, the rate of the second syringe may be increased. However, *do not* bolus the inotropes/vasopressor.

An example of a 'double-pumping' procedure is as follows:

- Step 1: Never leave the patient unattended.
- Step 2: Begin double pumping when there is at least 5 mL or 1 h worth of drug left in the current infusion syringe. Check the clamps are open to the first and second infusions.
- Step 3: Observe the patient's systolic BP to gauge a baseline BP.

- Step 4: Set the second syringe to run at the same rate as the first, that the first syringe is running, and then commence the infusion.
- Step 5: Observe the systolic BP until it rises by 10–20 mmHg, then begin to reduce the rate of the first syringe until it can be discontinued.
- Step 6: Continue to monitor the BP closely and if there is significant hypotension, inform the nurse in charge.
- Step 7: Replace the original syringe with a new one. However, drawing up the new infusion too far in advance may result in the drug becoming unstable.

It has to be stated that each critical care unit will have its own policies and protocols for the preparation and administration of double pumping, which must be adhered to.

Sepsis and shock due to COVID-19

COVID-19 is a viral infection and there is growing evidence that sepsis can be a complication [26]. Sepsis is not a specific illness, but a clinical syndrome characterized by severe inflammation, immunosuppression and altered activation of coagulation, in which every system in the body may be affected [27]. The revised international consensus definitions for sepsis describe it as [27,28]:

a life threatening organ dysfunction due a dysregulated host response to infection

and septic shock as [27,28]:

persisting hypotension requiring vasopressors to maintain a mean arterial pressure (MAP) of 65 mmHg or more and having a serum lactate level of greater than 2 mmol/l despite adequate volume resuscitation.

The Sequential (or Sepsis-related) Organ Failure Assessment (SOFA) score (Table 10.6) is a clinical criterion that predicts mortality in those infected patients most likely to have sepsis. The full SOFA score is not well known outside critical care and thus is not intended as a tool for patient management [31]. Each element contains a score of 1–4. The higher the number of points, the higher the risk of poor outcomes and mortality.

The quick SOFA (q-SOFA) (Table 10.7) score [32] is a modified, shorter version of the full SOFA score to identify those patients at risk of a poor outcome outside of critical care, where quick access to laboratory tests may not be available. This score contains three elements: altered mental status (Glasgow Coma Scale < 15), tachypnoea (>22 breaths per minute) and hypotension (systolic BP <100 mmHg). Each element is scored with a cumulative overall score. Two points or higher is associated with the onset of infection and is linked to a higher mortality rate. This score has been developed as a practical tool to identify those patients most at risk of death or a long critical care admission.

In COVID-19, it is generally accepted that SOFA is superior to q-SOFA [33]. However, Liu et al. [33] argued that either the SOFA or q-SOFA is effective as

TABLE 10.6 Sequential (or Sepsis-related) Organ Failure Assessment [29,30].

	Score				
	Organ dysfunction defined as a change of two or more points				
System	0	1	2	3	4
Respiration (PaO_2/FiO_2 mmHg) (kPa)	>400 (53.3)	<40 (53.3)	<300 (40)	<200 (26.7) with respiratory support	<100 (13.3) with respiratory support
Coagulation platelets ($\times 10^3/\mu L$)	>150	<150	<100	<50	<20
Liver bilirubin μmol/L (mg/dL)	<20 (1.2)	20–32 (1.2–1.9)	33–101 (2.0–5.9)	102–204 (6.0–11.9)	>204 (12.0)
Cardiovascular (catecholamine doses in μg/kg/min for at least 1 h)	MAP >70 mmHg	MAP <70 mmHg	Dopamine <5 or dobutamine (any dose)	Dopamine 5.1–15 or adrenaline <0.1 or noradrenaline <1	Dopamine >15 or adrenaline >0.1 or noradrenaline >0.1
Central nervous system (Glasgow Coma Scale)	15	13–14	10–12	6–9	<6
Renal creatinine μmol/L (mg/dL) Urine output (mL/day)	<110 (1.2)	110–170 (1.2–1.9)	171–299 (2.0–3.4)	300–440 (3.5–4.9) <500	>440 (5.0) <200

TABLE 10.7 q-Sequential (or Sepsis-related) Organ Failure Assessment criteria [27].

Respiratory rate >22/min
Altered mental state (Glasgow Coma Scale) <15
Systolic blood pressure <100 mmHg

an adjunct to risk stratification at admission for critically ill patients with suspected or confirmed COVID-19.

International consensus guidelines on the management of critically ill patients with COVID-19 identified the prevalence of shock in adult patients with COVID-19 ranging from 1% to 35% depending on the population studies, severity of illness and definition of shock [34]. The Surviving Sepsis Campaign international consensus guidelines suggest that in the absence of quality evidence of adults with COVID-19, shock dynamic parameters, including skin temperature, capillary refill time and/or serum lactate measurements over static parameters, should be used. The use of lactate levels to guide resuscitation is already accepted in sepsis treatment. When compared with central venous oxygen saturations, early lactate clearance-directed therapy was associated with a reduction in mortality, shorter ICU stay and shorter duration of mechanical ventilation [35].

Fluid resuscitation is complex in COVID-19 patients for preventing both pulmonary oedema due to ARDS and acute kidney injury. When fluid resuscitation is indicated, crystalloids over colloids are recommended, with starch, gelatin and dextran-based fluids being avoided [34]. In addition, it is suggested that the routine use of albumin for initial resuscitation be avoided [34].

For patients with suspected or confirmed COVID-19 who do not respond to fluid resuscitation, it is suggested that norepinephrine (noradrenaline) be used as the first-line vasoactive agent [34]. If norepinephrine is not available, vasopressin or epinephrine can be used; however, the evidence available is low quality [34]. Nevertheless, it is suggested that vasopressin should be used as a second-line agent over a titrating norepinephrine dose if MAP cannot be achieved with norepinephrine alone. Vasoactive agents need to be titrated to maintain a target MAP of 60–65 mmHg [34].

In COVID-19 patients with shock, evidence of cardiac dysfunction and persistent hypoperfusion, regardless of fluid status, the commencement of norepinephrine Dobutamine may be appropriate as an alternative to increasing norepinephrine infusions [34]. In refractory shock, the use of low-dose corticosteroid therapy may be beneficial; this may include a corticosteroid therapy regimen of intravenous hydrocortisone 200 mg per day either as an infusion or intermittent bolus [34].

Conclusion

Haemodynamic monitoring is an integral element of comprehensive nursing in critical care. COVID-19 is a complex disease and it has to be recognized that the systemic effects of COVID-19 on critically ill patients are still not fully known. It has to be recognized that not all patients will follow a standard disease trajectory and therefore nurses need to be flexible, adaptable and proactive in their response if they are to identify, interpret and respond to the rapid changes in patient status that accompany this pandemic. This chapter has given an overview of some of the key issues. It is the responsibility of every nurse to keep abreast of new developments in this rapidly changing and evolving pandemic.

References

[1] Michard F, Malbrain MLNG, Martin GS, Fumeaux T, Lobo S, Gonzalez F, Pinho-Oliveira V, Constantin JM. Haemodynamic monitoring and management in COVID-19 intensive care patients: an international survey. Anaesth Crit Care pain Med 2020. 39. 5. 563–569

[2] Haslam J, Ball J, Rhodes A, MacNaughton P. Chapter 3: monitoring. In: Nimmo GR, Singer M, editors. ABC of intensive care. 2nd ed. BMJ Books; 2011.

[3] Edwards S, Williams J. In: A nurse's survival guide to critical care. Elsevier; 2019. Updated.

[4] Resuscitation Council (UK). In: Advanced life support manual. 7th ed. 2016. [London].

[5] Hatchett R. Cardiac monitoring and the use of a systematic approach in interpreting electrocardiogram rhythms. Nurs Stand 2017;32(11):51–63.

[6] National Institute for Health and Care Excellence. Atrial fibrillation. 2020. https://cks.nice.org.uk/topics/atrial-fibrillation/.

[7] Kochi AN, Tagliari AP, Forleo GB, Fassini GM, Tondo C. Cardiac arrhythmic complications in patients with COVID-19. J Cardiovasc Electrophysiol 2020;31(5):1003–8.

[8] World Health Organisation. Coronavirus disease (COVID-19) advice for the public: Mythbusters. 2020. https://www.who.int/emergencies/diseases/novel-coronavirus-2019/advice-for-public/myth-busters.

[9] Morgan S. How to auscultate for heart sounds in adults. Nurs Stand 2017;32(5):41–3.

[10] Johnston-Walker E, Hardcastle J. Neurovascular assessment in the critically ill patient. Nurs Crit Care 2011;16(4). https://doi.org/10.1111/j.1478-5153.2011.00431.x.

[11] Klok FA, Kruip MJHA, van der Meer NJM, et al. Incidence of thrombotic complications in critically ill ICU patients with COVID-19. Thromb Res 2020. 191. 145–147

[12] Mayo P. Undertaking an accurate and comprehensive assessment of the acutely ill adult. Nurs Stand 2017;32(8):53–61.

[13] Ahern J, Philpot P. Assessing acutely ill patients on general wards. Nurs Stand 2002;16(47):47–54.

[14] Li Y, Jiao N, Zhu L, et al. Non-febrile COVID-19 patients were common and often became critically ill: a retrospective multicenter cohort study. Crit Care 2020;24:314.

[15] Wang D, Hu B, Hu C, Zhu F, Liu X, Zhang J, Wang B, Xiang H, Cheng Z, Xiong Y, et al. Clinical characteristics of 138 hospitalized patients with 2019 novel coronavirus-infected pneumonia in Wuhan, China. J Am Med Assoc 2020;323(11):1061–9.

[16] Huang C, Wang Y, Li X, Ren L, Zhao J, Hu Y, Zhang L, Fan G, Xu J, Gu X, et al. Clinical features of patients infected with 2019 novel coronavirus in Wuhan, China. Lancet 2020;395(10223):497–506.

[17] Goyal P, Choi JJ, Pinheiro LC, Schenck EJ, Chen R, Jabri A, Satlin MJ, Campion Jr TR, Nahid M, Ringel JB, et al. Clinical characteristics of COVID-19 in New York city. N Engl J Med 2020;382(24):2374.

[18] Richardson S, Hirsch JS, Narasimhan M, Crawford JM, McGinn T, Davidson KW, Northwell C-RC, Barnaby DP, Becker LB, Chelico JD, et al. Presenting characteristics, comorbidities, and outcomes among 5700 patients hospitalized with COVID-19 in the New York City area. J Am Med Assoc 2020;323(20):2052–9.

[19] Llitjos J-F, Leclerc M, Chochois C, et al. High incidence of venous thromboembolic events in anticoagulated severe COVID-19 patients. J Thromb Haemost 2020. 18. 7. 1743–1746

[20] Nahum J, Morichau-Beauchant T, Daviaud F, et al. Venous thrombosis among critically ill patients with coronavirus disease 2019 (COVID-19). JAMA Netw Open 2020;3(5). e2010478.

[21] Harvey S, Harrison DA, Singer M, Ashcroft J, Jones CM, Elbourne D, Brampton W, Williams D, Young D, Rowan K. Assessment of the clinical effectiveness of pulmonary artery catheters in management of patients in intensive care (PAC-Man): a randomized controlled trial. Lancet 2005;366:472–7.

[22] Becker D, Franges EZ, Geiter H, et al. Critical care nursing made incredibly easy. Lippincott Williams and Wilkins; 2004.

[23] Parry A. Inotropic drugs and their uses in critical care. Nurs Crit Care 2011;17(1):19–27.

[24] Koczmara C, St-Arnaud C, Martines HQ, Adhikari NKJ, Meade MO, Berard D, Leclair MA, Hyland S, Torres E, Fontaine L, Beland F, Martel A, Samson S, Dubreuil J, Lageueux G, Lamarre P, Langevin C, Lamontagne F. Vasopressor stewardship: a case report and lessons shared. Dynamics 2014;25(1):26–9.

[25] Cox J, Roche S. Vasopressors and development of pressure ulcers in adult critical care. Am J Crit Care 2015;24(6):501–10.

[26] Sepsis.org. The connection between COVID-19 sepsis and sepsis survivors. 2020. https://www.sepsis.org/news/the-connection-between-covid-19-sepsis-and-sepsis-survivors/.

[27] Singer M, et al. The third international consensus definitions for sepsis and septic shock (Sepsis-3). J Am Med Assoc 2016;315(8):801–10. https://doi.org/10.1001/jama.2016.0287.

[28] NICE. Sepsis: recognition, diagnosis and early management. 2016. www.nice.org.uk/guidance/ng51/resources/sepsis-recognition-diagnosis-and-early-management-1837508256709.

[29] Rhodes A, Evans LE, Alhazzani W, et al. Surviving Sepsis Campaign: international guidelines for management of sepsis and septic shock: 2016. Intensive Care Med 2017;43(3):304–77.

[30] British Medical Journal. Sepsis in adults: Criteria. 2020. https://bestpractice.bmj.com/topics/en-gb/3000098/criteria.

[31] Vincent J, Martin GS, Levy MM. qSOFA does not replace SIRS in the definition of sepsis. Crit Care 2016;20:210.

[32] Seymour CW, Liu VX, Iwashyna TJ, Brunkhorst FM, Rea TD, Scherag A, et al. Assessment of clinical criteria for sepsis: for the third international consensus definitions for sepsis and septic shock (Sepsis-3). J Am Med Assoc. 315. 762–774.

[33] Liu S, Yao N, Qiu Y, He C. Predictive performance of SOFA and qSOFA for in-hospital mortality in severe novel coronavirus disease. Am J Emerg Med 2020. https://doi.org/10.1016/j.ajem.2020.07.019. 2020. 38. 10. 2074–2080.

[34] Alhazzani W, Moller MH, Arabi YM, Loeb M, Gong MNN, Fan E, Oczkowshi S, Levy MM, Derde L, Dzierba A, et al. Surviving sepsis campaign: guidelines on the management of critically ill adults with coronavirus disease 2019 (COVID-19). Crit Care Med 2020;48(6):E440–69.

[35] Pan J, Peng M, Liao C, et al. Relative efficacy and safety of early lactate clearance-guided therapy resuscitation in patients with sepsis: a meta-analysis. Medicine (Baltimore) 2019;98:e14453.

Chapter 11

Acute kidney injury

Chris Carter, Janice Ferreira, Babita Gurung, Joy Notter

Chapter Outline

Acute kidney injury (AKI) is described as a rapid decline in renal function over a 48-h period, leading to an inability to maintain fluid, electrolyte and acid–base balance [1,2]. It has been identified as a common complication of critical illness, with an estimated prevalence of 25%–65% [3]. Elsayed [4] reported a 6.3% incidence of severe AKI during the first 24 h of ICU admission, with AKI accounting for 9.3% of all ICU bed days. In severe COVID-19 disease there is a raised incidence of AKI and renal injury in approximately 20%–35% of critically ill patients [5]. The cause was initially thought to be due to the effects of acute respiratory failure. However, it is now thought that the systemic effects of COVID-19 cause multiple system organ failure (MSOF) and complications arising from other risk factors such as age, diabetes mellitus, cardiovascular disease, hypertension, vasopressor medications and the need for non-invasive and invasive ventilation [6,7]. There is increasing evidence that members of the Black, Asian and minority ethnic (BAME) communities are at greater risk of complications from COVID-19 [8]. For all patients AKI is recognized as being one of the key causes of increased morbidity, poor prognosis and mortality, with recent evidence indicating that over 50% of the group develop AKI within 24 h of intubation and invasive ventilation [6]. In consequence, critical care nurses have a responsibility to closely monitor renal function, recognizing and responding early to prevent the progression and severity of AKI.

COVID-19: A Critical Care Textbook. https://doi.org/10.1016/B978-0-7020-8383-9.00011-7

Anatomy and physiology of renal function and fluid balance

The renal system is responsible for the removal of metabolic waste, maintaining fluid balance and electrolytes, acid–base homeostasis, blood pressure, red blood cell production and hormone balance [9]. Therefore, any reduction in activity and function will have a systemic impact on fluid balance and homeostasis [10]. Any reduction in circulating plasma volume affects cellular oxygenation, which triggers compensatory mechanisms to restore homeostasis. A reduction in blood pressure causes a series of renal, neural and adrenergic responses and triggers the secretion of renin by the kidneys into the bloodstream, which in turn activates the renin–angiotensin–aldosterone system (RAAS) pathway. This then promotes the adrenal cortex to secrete aldosterone (hormone), which causes the renal tubules to increase the reabsorption of sodium, releasing water back into the circulatory system, increasing plasma volume and blood pressure. In addition, as aldosterone regulates potassium levels, an increase in the extracellular fluid causes a rise in aldosterone levels, resulting in additional potassium ions being excreted via the kidneys in the urine, so maintaining the electrolyte balance in the body.

Additional compensatory mechanisms include vasoconstriction following the release of renin, which converts angiotensinogen to angiotensin I. This is then converted into angiotensin II by angiotensin-converting enzyme (ACE), which is secreted by the vascular endothelium, particularly in the lungs. Angiotensin II is a powerful vasoconstrictor, resulting in a blood pressure increase. Plasma volume is further regulated by antidiuretic hormone (ADH), secreted by the posterior pituitary gland, when osmoreceptors and baroreceptors detect a decrease in osmolarity and blood pressure. Normally, this results in increased thirst, an early warning indicator of altered fluid body volume. In critical care settings, the patient's fluid balance, biochemistry and systemic observations are regularly monitored and recorded to detect complications.

Classification of AKI

The AKI criteria have evolved in recent years, with diagnosis now based on monitoring serum creatinine (sCr) levels, with or without an adequate urine output. This current diagnostic approach is based on an acute decrease in the glomerular filtration rate (GFR) with an acute increase in sCr levels over a specific period of time, which may be accompanied by a decline in urine output [11]. Mortality due to AKI varies considerably and is determined by severity, clinical setting and other patient-related factors. In the UK, AKI is largely preventable, with mortality varying between 25% and 30% [12]. In critical care, an estimated 5% of patients will go on to require RRT [1,2,4]. Causes of AKI can be identified by three categories, pre-, intra- or post-renal condition (Table 11.1) [1,13,14]. If untreated it will eventually escalate to renal cellular damage and ultimately intrinsic renal disease [11,14].

TABLE 11.1 Causes of AKI [1,13,14].

Prerenal	Hypovolaemia, e.g., haemorrhage, gastrointestinal losses, excessive diuresis, and third spacing (ascites, pancreatitis) Hypotension and low cardiac output states, e.g., myocardial dysfunction, arrhythmias Sepsis
Intrarenal	Hepatorenal syndrome Cortical necrosis Acute tubular necrosis, e.g., nephrotoxins (e.g., radiographic contrast, aminoglycosides, rhabdomyolysis). Acute interstitial nephritis – drugs including penicillins and NSAIDs Vascular, e.g., emboli.
Post-renal	Raised intra-abdominal pressure causing reduced renal venous drainage Intraureteral conditions – calculi, tumour, blood clot Extraureteral conditions – retroperitoneal fibrosis, tumour, aneurysm Bladder obstruction – prostatic hypertrophy, bladder tumour, blood clot, calculi, functional neuropathy Urethral obstruction

Prerenal

Severe COVID-19 can cause several prerenal complications due to prolonged periods of fever, excessive perspiration, increased work of breathing, gastric losses and self-starvation of fluids due to lack of appetite and lethargy. In consequence, patients may present with a significant deficit in fluid balance from insensible losses, causing them to be intravascularly dehydrated. Therefore, insensible losses should be factored into fluid balance assessment and management. Previous management of limiting fluid intake to prevent severe acute respiratory distress syndrome (ARDS) has been disproven in COVID-19 [15]. Instead, fluid balance interventions must be continually adjusted in the light of patient responsiveness. In severe COVID-19, there may be delayed-onset AKI at between 11 and 20 days post-infection [2].

The effect of positive-pressure ventilation and the use of positive end-expiratory pressure (PEEP) may increase intrathoracic pressures, decrease cardiac output and increase right ventricular afterload. This impairs right ventricular function, which detrimentally increases the systemic nervous pressure, reducing renal perfusion and increasing venous congestion. High tidal volumes lead to increased release of pro-inflammatory mediators and therefore, lung-protective strategies are crucial to reduce cytokine burden and organ dysfunction [16]. Treatment for ARDS may include maintaining a neutral fluid balance as long as this does not adversely affect other organs. This may include the use of diuretics to achieve fluid balance, however, the risk/benefit ratio and an individual patient assessment must be considered. Strategies to improve oxygenation, including the prone position, may contribute to low cardiac output, reduction of gastric motility, increased intra-abdominal pressure and oedema of the digestive system. Any or all of these can contribute to increase renal artery pressure constricting circulation to the kidneys. To protect renal function, continuous sedation used to facilitate ventilator synchrony has to be carefully considered [17], with propofol and dexmedetomidine associated with lower risk of AKI development, when compared with longer acting sedatives [16].

Intrarenal

Potential intrarenal complications may be due to the profound hypoxaemia and respiratory failure caused by severe COVID-19. As part of the immune system response to infections, cytokines (small proteins) are released. However, this sudden influx causes a severe systemic inflammation response, leading to damage of healthy tissue. This pathway increases renal tubular injury, due to virus replication processes and systemic hypoperfusion [18]. It is accepted that COVID-19 relies on ACE2 and transmembrane serine proteases (TMPRSS) cells as a form of entry and replication within the human body [19]. In patients with a high viral load, the severity of renal failure may be higher, due to the accumulation of virus in the kidney tubules [7,18]. Given the effects on the renal system, COVID-19 is likely to be present in urine samples, making it essential that strict infection prevention and control strategies are followed when handling all bodily fluids. Other potential complications include the development of microthrombosis, causing obstruction at a cellular level and preventing oxygen moving between the circulating volume and cells of organs, which can lead to acute tubular necrosis and organ dysfunction [2].

Post-renal

Post-renal complications may be exacerbated in patients with urinary system conditions, for example, enlarged prostate. Iatrogenic complications include blocked urinary catheters or kinked urinary catheter tubing.

Guidelines for practice

The Kidney Disease Improving Global Outcomes (KDIGO) [20] guidelines were developed to guide fluid balance. In critical care, the dynamic changing status is evidenced by alterations in cardiac or respiratory systems which indicate improvement or deterioration of renal function and other systems. KDIGO provides a framework for the classification of AKI (Diagram 11.1). An AKI is defined as an increase in serum creatinine (SCr) by ≥ 0.3 mg/dL (≥ 26.5 μmol/L) within 48h; or increase in sCr to ≥ 1.5 times baseline, which is known or presumed to have occurred within the prior 7 days; or urine volume <0.5 mL/kg/h for 6h (Table 11.2).

AKI Causes and Stages

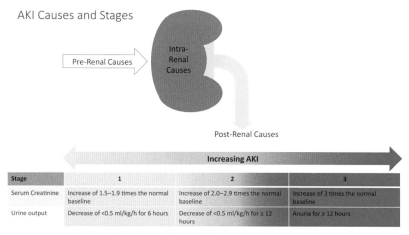

DIAGRAM 11.1 AKI causes and stages.

TABLE 11.2 KDIGO criteria and staging of AKI [20].

Stage	Serum creatinine		Urine output
1	Increase of 1.5–1.9 times the normal baseline	Increase of ≥0.3 mg/dL (≥26.5 µmol/L)	Decrease of <0.5 mL/kg/h for 6 h
2	Increase of 2.0–2.9 times the normal baseline		Decrease of <0.5 mL/kg/h for≥12 h
3	Increase of 3 times the normal baseline	Increase of ≥4 mg/dL (≥353.6 µmol/L)	Anuria for≥12 h

In critical care settings, most patients will have hourly accurate fluid balance, including cumulative balances, recorded. However, it has to be noted that maintaining optimal fluid balance may be hard to achieve, as calculating insensible losses, for example tachypnoea and fever, may be challenging. Urinary catheter care should include checking of the colour of urine and for any signs of debris, checking the catheter site and prevention of the catheter dragging or pulling on the urethra. In addition, urinary output should be monitored hourly, the amount of urine produced is based on actual body weight, with a target of greater than 0.5 mL/kg/h. Decisions on the frequency of monitoring of serum creatinine, urea and creatinine kinase are dependent upon the patient's condition and should take account of therapeutic monitoring and the use of nephrotoxic drugs [16].

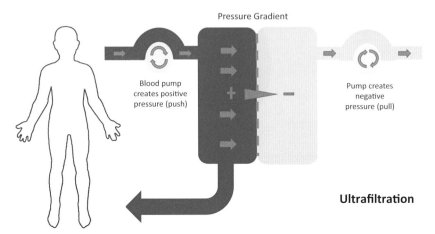

DIAGRAM 11.2   Positive/negative pressure gradient.

Using the KDIGO guidelines, initiation of CRRT in AKI should be based on individual clinical assessment. Indications for initiating treatment include metabolic acidosis (pH > 6.5), hyperkalaemia (7.6 mmol/L), fluid overload, toxicity (drugs, poisons and toxic compounds), severe uraemic symptoms, urea >30 mmol/L and rising, creatinine >300 mmol/L and rising, oliguria for 12 h (30 mL/h for 6 h, not responding to diuretics or haemodynamic optimization), hyperthermia, persistently high lactate associated with metabolic acidosis and clinically significant organ oedema.

CRRT involves blood being passed through an extracorporeal circuit from a special vascular catheter (VasCath). The speed of the blood flow is controlled by a roller pump, the blood is then passed through a semipermeable polysulphone membrane, which contains multiple fibres with pores. The size of the pores determines the substances (molecule size) that can pass through, allowing the movement of waste products but maintaining the cells and other blood proteins in the intravascular compartment. This is referred to as ultrafiltration, a positive to negative pressure gradient is used, which results in fluid passing through the membrane from the blood side to the dialysate (filtration fluid) (Diagram 11.2). For this process to be effective the hydrostatic pressure in the blood has to be higher than the pressure in the ultrafiltrate, to allow plasma water with solutes to cross the membrane (termed 'solute drag'). The faster the flow rate, the higher the clearance. Medium-sized molecules are cleared by convection, a one-way movement of solutes, while smaller molecules are removed by diffusion. Following the movement of particles from higher concentration (blood side) to lower concentration (dialysate), blood is then returned to the patient via the second port of the VasCath [21]. Anticoagulant is used to reduce the risk of clot formation within the extracorporeal circuit. Anticoagulation may be provided systemically or regionally. Types of anticoagulation include regional

Types of CRRT Modalities

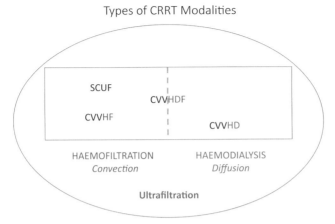

DIAGRAM 11.3   Types of treatment modalities.

citrate, heparin and, on occasion, prostacyclin. International consensus guidelines recommend the use of regional citrate, however, nurses need to be aware of the potential serious side effects and must closely monitor all patients [20,22].

There are several types of RRT modalities (Diagram 11.3), these include continuous arteriovenous haemo(dia)filtration (CAVH/D), this first-generation development of RRT is rarely used in practice today [23]. Slow continuous ultrafiltration (SCUF) is regulated by gravity or pump and generates ultrafiltrate. Continuous venovenous haemofiltration (CVVHF) involves a pump generating a hydrostatic pressure, with ultrafiltrate produced. Continuous venovenous haemodialysis (CVVHD) involves dialysate fluid being added to the haemofilter and a pump using convention to move dialysate. Continuous venovenous haemodiafiltration (CVVHDF) is a combination of both CAVHF and CVVHD, and is deemed the most effective and most frequently used [24].The choice of treatment modality depends on the needs of the patient and physician preference.

Disadvantages of CRRT include that only one patient at a time can be treated per session, and sessions can last for days. Patients with severe COVID-19 disease may also develop hypercoagulation, which may require systemic anticoagulation, in consequence, there is an increased risk of extracorporeal membranes clotting. This may lead to additional time and resources for trouble-shooting and repriming filters. In addition, there may be delays in treatment and potential worsening of condition.

Peritoneal dialyses (PD) is a form of RRT whereby dialysate is administered directly into the peritoneal cavity by gravity, remaining for a short period of time to allow diffusion, osmosis and ultrafiltration before drainage. This therapy was developed in 1920 but only recognized as lifesaving therapy in 1946 [25]. Although rarely used in the critical care setting as it has been superseded by other forms of renal replacement therapies, the impact of a pandemic such as

COVID-19 may result in it being reinstituted in situations when other forms of CRRT are oversubscribed or not available [25].

Advantages to using PD include that there are no clotting concerns as no anticoagulation of circuits is required. Patients do not require a VasCath, decreasing the risk of line-associated bloodstream infections. Disadvantages include that the procedure cannot be performed if the patient is in the prone position, and it is contraindicated in patients with recent abdominal surgery, abdominal adhesions, peritonitis or pregnancy. There is also no control over the rate of fluid removal. Specialist trained staff with technical expertise are required for catheter insertion and ongoing care.

Nursing practice

In some settings, specialist renal nurses focus on the care of patients receiving CRRT, allowing the critical care nurse to focus on other aspects of patient care [26]. However, in countries such as the UK, the critical care nurse's role is to start, monitor, assess and discontinue therapy [24]. Caring for a critically ill patient requiring RRT can be daunting, with careful monitoring an essential part of the nurse's role because CRRT may potentiate hypotension, arrhythmias, membrane bio-incompatibility, complications of vascular access and anticoagulation administration challenges, in addition to monitoring patient management and recognition of complications. These include thrombus formation within the extracorporeal circuit, which impacts adversely on treatment and can result in iatrogenic blood loss due to loss of circuits, with a concomitant need for blood transfusions and increased financial costs arising from the high usage of circuits [27,28]. In recognition of this, extracorporeal circuits are anticoagulated to maintain patency. Commonly used anticoagulants include heparin, prostacyclin, regional citrate and/or thrombin [24].

In addition to these issues, patient management includes the prevention of infection or transmission of infection, and seeking problems arising from treatment. This can include low access pressure, high or low return pressure, high transmembrane pressure (TMP), high filter pressure, air detection in the circuit, blood leak and issues with fluid balance and scales.

To facilitate CRRT, VasCaths are used to access and keep patent the central venous lines necessary. These have two wide-bore lumens which allow for faster flow than standard central lines, with the length differing for neck (15 cm) and femoral (20 cm) routes. It has to be noted that the location of the VasCath is critical to success, as poor access may lead to inadequate blood flow and increased risk of filter circuits clotting [21]. The preferred locations are outlined in Table 11.3.

During the insertion of the VasCath, the role of the nurse is to assist the medical team, to provide reassurance to patients that are awake and to monitor the patient for complications, for example, arrhythmias or tension pneumothorax. Other potential complications include artery puncture, lacerations of the vena cava, mediastinal vessels and right atrium; haematoma formation

TABLE 11.3 Hierarchy of choice for VasCath insertion [21].

- First choice: right internal jugular.
- Second choice: femoral vein
- Third choice: left internal jugular
- Fourth choice: subclavian

including haemothorax; catheter entanglement can occur in patients with multiple catheters, pneumothorax, tracheal injury, air embolus and/or subcutaneous emphysema.

Strict aseptic techniques must be followed when inserting or handling these lines. When not in use, VasCaths tend to be 'locked' with an anticoagulant to prevent clot formation. In many settings, 10 mL of blood is aspirated from each lumen before flushing the line and attaching the CRRT lines. Before attaching the patient to the filter, the team needs to confirm the position of the VasCath. For example, a chest X-ray is essential if the line is inserted in either the jugular or subclavian veins.

A low or high access pressure may occur when the VasCath becomes juxtaposed with a vessel wall or becomes partially or fully clotted. It may also occur if the lumen or lines become kinked or clamped. Some common potential solutions including checking both lumens and tubing are straight and unclamped. Where problems arise, the VasCath and CRRT lines should be checked to ascertain that the VasCath is correctly positioned (e.g., sutured in place and has not moved position). The patient's fluid balance needs to be continuously monitored, as a negative fluid balance can indicate the patient may be intravascularly depleted, which will cause the veins to collapse. Aspiration of both VasCath lumens followed by flushing with normal saline indicates whether or not there may be formation of clots within the VasCath, and if so which one is blocked. Limb positions must be checked as bent legs or neck position (for example, if a femoral catheter and patient has his leg bent, this may cause suction against the femoral wall). Machine malfunctions may occur, therefore, spare equipment including a replacement CRRT should be available.

Where a low return pressure is identified checks should be made that the low blood pump speed has not fallen or return tubing become disconnected. Patients on long-term dialysis may be given a VasCath for temporary CRRT when or if they are transferred into a critical care setting. To reduce this risk all connections should be checked, and this includes ascertaining that the VasCath has not migrated resulting in exposure of the return port.

A rapid rise in the transmembrane pressure (TMP) is a cause for concern, and may arise from filtrate tubing or bags being occluded by a clamp or kinking. A high TMP at the start of treatment may indicate the ratio of pressure between the blood flow and replacement fluid is too high (the overall flow is too rapid). A slow rise in TMP may suggest that the extracorporeal circuit is slowly clotting. Where this is suspected, verification of the presence of a clot within the filter may indicate the need to electively change the circuit.

High prefilter pressure may be caused by kinked tubing, a clot forming in the return chamber or the circuit. Nurses need to check the tubing is straight, and where high pressures continue, they should consider predilution on the next CRRT cycle. Incorrect assembly and management of CRRT may result in complications such as air being detected in the circuit, the circuit being incorrectly positioned in the CRRT machine causing blood leak or dialysate fluid being incorrectly hung or remain clamped. In consequence, in many units, checklists have been developed and hourly observation of patient CRRT parameters are recorded, including error checks.

The decision to discontinue therapy will be based on patient parameters and the ongoing patient condition and response to treatment. For most patients the intrinsic recovery of the kidneys allows them to return to function without the CRRT support, the markers for this will rely on urine creatinine clearance (>15 mL/min), stable sCr without CRRT, urine output and gradual weaning from CRRT.

Conclusion

Evidence from local, national and international statistics indicates that AKI is a common complication of severe COVID-19 disease. The nurse is the only healthcare professional permanently at the bedside of patients and, therefore, is in a position to recognize AKI early, to respond to the signs, initiating treatment and referring to specialist help where appropriate. The window of opportunity for treatment in COVID-19 is short, nevertheless evidence from recent epicentres arising from the first wave of COVID-19 has revealed that a rapid response from nurses can improve patient outcomes. It has to be accepted that the unprecedented numbers seeking treatment during a pandemic are such that pressure on CRRT resources can limit access to treatment for all. Where this occurs the outcomes for all COVID-19 patients will be adversely affected.

References

[1] Baid H, Creed F, Hargreaves J. Oxford handbook of critical care nursing. Oxford University Press; 2016.

[2] Selby NM, Forni LG, Laing CM, Horne KL, Evans RDR, Lucas BJ, Fluck RJ. Covid-19 and acute kidney injury in hospital: summary of NICE guidelines. Br Med J 2020;369:m1963. https://doi.org/10.1136/bmj.m196.

[3] Albarran J. Chapter 2: Epidemiology and pathogenesis of AKI. In: Albarran JW, Saraiva M, editors. Acute kidney injury: a guide to clinical practice. European Dialysis and Transplant Nurses Association/European Renal Care Association (EDTNA/ERCA); 2012.

[4] Elsayed I, Pawley N, Rosser J, Heap MJ, Mills GH, Tridente A, Raithatha AH. Survival outcomes and length of stay in acute kidney injury patients receiving renal replacement therapy on intensive care in a UK teaching hospital: a comparison of ethnicity, age and gender demographic data. Crit Care 2015;19(Suppl. 1):305.

[5] Intensive Care Society. COVID-19: a synthesis of clinical experience in UK intensive care settings. 2020. [London].

[6] Jhaveri K, Meir L, Flores Chang B, Parikh R, Wanchoo R, Barilla-LaBarca M, Bijol V, Hajizadeh N. Thrombotic micro angiopathy in a patient with COVID-19. Kidney Int 2020;98(2):509–12.

[7] Pan XW, Xu D, Zhang H, Zhou W, Wang LH, Cui XG. Identification of a potential mechanism of acute kidney injury during the COVID-19 outbreak: a study based on single-cell transcriptome analysis. Intensive Care Med 2020;46(6):114–6. https://doi.org/10.1007/s00134-020-06026-1.

[8] Raisi-Estabragh Z, McCracken C, Bethell MS, Cooper J, Cooper C, Caulfield MJ, Munroe PB, Harvey NC, Petersen SE. Greater risk of severe COVID-19 in Black, Asian and Minority Ethnic populations is not explained by cardio metabolic, socioeconomic or behavioural factors, or by 25(OH)-vitamin D status: study of 1326 cases from the UK Biobank. J Public Health 2020;42(3):451–60.

[9] Andrade M, Knight J. Anatomy and physiology of ageing 4: the renal system. Nurs Times 2017;113(5):46–9.

[10] McLafferty E, Johnstone C, Hendry C, et al. Fluid and electrolyte balance. Nurs Stand 2014;28(29):42–9.

[11] Makris K, Spanou L. Acute kidney injury: definition, pathophysiology and clinical phenotypes. Clin Biochem Rev 2016;37(2):85–98.

[12] Ftouh S, Thomas M. Acute kidney injury: summary of NICE guidance. BMJ 2013;347(2):4930.

[13] Edwards S, Williams J, editors. A nurse's survival guide to critical care. Elsevier; 2019. Updated.

[14] National Institute for Health and Care Excellence. Acute kidney injury: what causes it?. 2018. https://cks.nice.org.uk/topics/acute-kidney-injury/.

[15] Ronco C, Reis T, Husain-Syed F. Management of acute kidney injury in patients with COVID-19. Lancet Respir Med 2020;8(7):738–42.

[16] Joannidis M, Forni LG, Klein SJ, et al. Lung-kidney interactions in critically ill patients: consensus report of the Acute Disease Quality Initiative (ADQI) 21 Workgroup. Intens Care Med 2020;46:654–72.

[17] Hanidziar D, Bittner EA. Sedation of mechanically ventilated COVID-19 patients: challenges and special considerations. Anaesth Analges 2020;131(1):e40–1. https://doi.org/10.1213/ANE.0000000000004887.

[18] Bo D, Chenhui W, Rongshuai W, Zeqing F, Yingjun T, Huiming W, Changsong W, Liang L, Ying L, Yueping L, Gang W, Zilin Y, Liang R, Yuzhang W, Yongwen C. Human kidney is a target for novel severe acute respiratory syndrome coronavirus 2 (SARS-CoV-2) infection. medRxiv 2020;3:4.

[19] Ward P. COVID-19/SARS-CoV-2 pandemic. Faculty of Pharmaceutical Medicine Blog; 2020. Available from: https://www.fpm.org.uk/blog/covid-19-sars-cov-2-pandemic/.

[20] KDIGO. Clinical practice guideline for acute kidney injury. Kidney international supplement. 2012. www.kdigo.org.

[21] Gemmell L, Docking R. Renal replacement therapy in critical care. BJA Educ 2017;17(3):88–93.

[22] Deep A, Zoha M, Dutta Kukreja P. Prostacyclin as an anticoagulant for continuous renal replacement therapy in children. Blood Purif 2017;43(4):279–89. https://doi.org/10.1159/000452754.

[23] OussamaRifai A, Murad LB, Sekkarie MA, Al-Makki AA, Zanabli AR, Kayal AA, Soudan KA. Continuous venovenous hemofiltration using a stand-alone blood pump for acute kidney injury in field hospitals in Syria. Kidney Int 2020;87(2):254–61.

[24] Richardson A, Whatmore J. Nursing essential principles: continuous renal replacement therapy. Nurs Crit Care 2014;20:8–14.

[25] Cullis B, Abdelraheem M, Abrahams G, Balbi A, Cruz DN, Frishberg Y, Koch V, McCulloch M, Numanoglu A, Nourse P, Pecoits-Filho R, Ponce D, Warady B, Yeates K, Finkelstein FO. Peritoneal dialysis for acute kidney injury. Perit Dial Int 2014;34(5):494–517. https://doi.org/10.3747/pdi.2013.00222.

[26] Ricci Z, Benelli S, Barbarigo F, Cocozza G, Pettinelli N, Di Luca E, Mettifogo M, Toniolo A, Ronco C. Nursing procedures during continuous renal replacement therapies: a national survey. Heart Lung Vessel 2015;7(3):224–30. PMID: 26495268; PMCID: PMC4593015.

[27] Tillman J. Heparin versus citrate for anticoagulation in critically ill patients treated with continuous renal replacement therapy. Nurs Crit Care 2009;14(4):191–9.

[28] Bai M, Zhou M, He L, Ma F, Li Y, Yu Y, Wang P, Li L, Jing R, Zhao L, Sun S. Citrate versus heparin anticoagulation for continuous renal replacement therapy: an updated meta-analysis of RCTs. Intens Care Med 2015;41(12):2098–110. https://doi.org/10.1007/s00134-015-4099-0. PMID: 26482411.

Chapter 12

Neurological care, sedation and pain management

Chris Carter, Joy Notter

Chapter Outline

Assessing the neurological status of a patient is a core component of critical care nursing. In COVID-19, the rapid onset of symptoms and increased severity result in the window of opportunity for treatment being time limited. An incomplete assessment can result in changes in signs and symptoms being missed, which in turn delays treatment for potentially life-threatening conditions. Treatment regimens must be based on evidence, compiled during a comprehensive assessment and regular systematic monitoring and evaluation. The nature of critical care treatments is complex and complicated, and it has to be accepted that individual patient response varies in terms of both onset and severity. Nurses need to have the knowledge and expertise to recognize early signs of fluctuating changes in neurological status. However, the staffing implications arising in the COVID-19 pandemic are such that staff are being redeployed to critical care with differing levels of experience in managing patients' altered conscious levels and receiving a combination of pharmacological interventions. Qualified critical care nurses may find themselves supervising a group of newly deployed staff who, while delivering direct patient care, will need mentoring and guidance to maintain patient safety. Therefore this chapter explores the principles of neurological assessment and nursing care of a patient receiving a continuous sedation, analgesia and/or neuromuscular blocking agent. Many of the patients with COVID-19 have existing co-morbidities, which may include undetected neurological impairments impacting on outcomes. Balancing all these factors is challenging, demanding and can be daunting for nurses adjusting to a new and rapidly changing environment.

COVID-19: A Critical Care Textbook. https://doi.org/10.1016/B978-0-7020-8383-9.00012-9

TABLE 12.1 Glasgow Coma Scale.

Eyes	4. Spontaneous
	3. To sound
	2. To pressure
	1. None
Verbal response	5. Orientated
	4. Confused
	3. Words
	2. Sounds
	1. None
Motor response	6. Obey commands
	5. Localizing
	4. Normal flexion
	3. Abnormal flexion
	2. Extension
	1. None

The speed at which the pandemic developed meant that little had been published on the use of sedation and analgesia for COVID-19 patients [1]. However, with the large numbers of patients requiring mechanical ventilation and the subsequent need for sedation and analgesia infusions, this is a cause for concern, as it poses several challenges for practice [1]. Health professionals need access to research and education regarding prescribing and using sedation, analgesia and neuromuscular blocking agents. Without guidance there is a risk of over- and/or underuse. As COVID-19 is a new disease, it is essential that good practice is shared to standardize care provision.

Neurological assessment

It is recognized that COVID-19 patients may be agitated, confused or poorly responsive [2]. In addition, conscious patients with suspected or confirmed COVID-19 are at risk of rapid deterioration, loss of consciousness and partial or full airway compromise, because individuals lose the ability to protect their own airway. Therefore neurological assessment should include use of the Glasgow Coma Scale (GCS) and pupil reaction. The GCS (Table 12.1) is a 15-point scale to monitor level of consciousness by patient responses: eye, verbal and motor. Scores should be recorded for each response and may suggest severe impairment (coma)=3–8, moderate impairment=9–12 or mild impairment=13–15. Neurological assessment should take account of the effects of drugs and underlying causes and interventions; for example, in ventilated patients, a 'T' may be used to signify tube.

Advantages of the GCS include its ease of use and no special equipment is needed. As it is widely used, the majority of staff are familiar with its design (it is already incorporated into some critical care observation charts) and it is a good predictor of outcome. However, disadvantages are that it is poor at monitoring changes

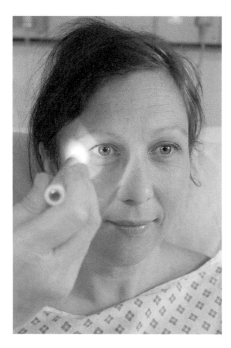

PICTURE 12.1 Using a pen torch to assess pupillary reaction.

in levels of consciousness and it is unreliable in middle range scores. Accuracy in estimating pupil size and assessing motor weakness varies between staff. Also, the type and location used to assess response to painful stimuli can vary (peripheral vs. central). Therefore, where possible the same assessor should complete the score. During handover, there should be a shared assessment by the departing and oncoming nurse.

Assessing pupillary reaction is an important component of the GCS assessment. When checking the pupils, a pen torch should be used (Picture 12.1). The average pupil size is 2–6 mm, but varies according to the time of day and the amount of light available. Both pupils should be identical in size and react equally to light. The intensity of the reaction, that is, whether brisk, sluggish or absent, should be noted (Picture 12.2). It is important to note if the patient has a pre-existing abnormality or irregularity of the eye(s), for example, cataracts, which will affect the response. In addition, it is important to note any drugs or medications the patients may have had. Some cause dilation (e.g., atropine), while others (opiates, e.g., morphine) cause constriction. Prosthetic eyes will not elicit a pupillary response. The size of pupillary assessment and reaction should be documented as per local policy and guidelines [3].

Sedation

Until the late 1990s it was accepted practice that patients requiring mechanical ventilation were heavily sedated and/or paralyzed; this changed when evidence demonstrated the negative outcome of deep sedation [4]. During the COVID-19 pandemic it was reported that, in some units, a return to deeper sedation was used to

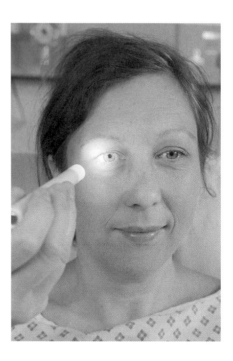

PICTURE 12.2 Pupil reaction.

prevent the risk of self-extubation, given the high risk of performing an emergency re-intubation and the risk of exposure to COVID-19 for the healthcare team [1]. This, together with less-than-ideal staff-to-patient ratios and a reduction in trained critical care staff providing direct patient care, has to be a cause for concern [5].

With a more lightly sedated ventilated patient, there is the possibility for a greater degree of interaction between the patient and the nurse, helping to promote person-centred care [6]. However, both sedated and non-sedated patients requiring ventilation may experience feelings of vulnerability, anxiousness, fear and loneliness [6]. Finding a balance between appropriate sedation and avoiding oversedation is complex, varying between patients. Nurse-driven sedation scales such as the Richmond Agitation and Sedation Score (RASS) (Table 12.2) allow the nurse to objectively assess a patient's sedation and titrate the medication accordingly. It is important to state that sedation, analgesia and paralyzing agents are *not* one and the same thing. While some analgesics and anxiolytics sedate (and vice versa), the indications for use are different [7,8].

If using intravenous sedation, this should be titrated based on RASS. Table 12.3 provides an example of how to titrate sedation infusions. While lighter sedation (RASS of 0 to −2) is appropriate for many ventilated patients, those requiring neuromuscular blocking agents will require a deeper level of sedation (RASS −4 to −5).

Patients with severe COVID-19 may require higher doses of sedation and analgesia, as well as multiple combinations of agents to facilitate critical care

TABLE 12.2 Richmond Agitation and Sedation Score [7].

+4	Combative	Overtly combative, violent, immediate danger to staff
+3	Very agitated	Pulls or removes tube(s) or catheter(s), aggressive
+2	Agitated	Frequent non-purposeful movement, fights ventilator
+1	Restless	Anxious but movements not aggressive, vigorous
0	Alert and calm	
−1	Drowsy	Not fully alert, but has sustained awakening (eye opening/eye contact) to voice (>10s)
−2	Light sedation	Briefly awakens with eye contact to voice (<10s)
−3	Moderate sedation	Movement or eye opening to voice (but no eye contact)
−4	Deep sedation	No response to voice, but movement or eye opening to physical stimulation
−5	Unarousable	No response to voice or physical stimulation

TABLE 12.3 Example titration of sedation based on Richmond Agitation and Sedation Score (RASS).

RASS	Action
+4	Bolus and increase infusion by 40%
+3	Bolus and increase infusion by 30%
+2	Bolus and increase infusion by 20%
+1	Bolus and increase infusion by 10%
0	No change
−1	No change
−2	Reduce infusion by 20%
−3	Reduce infusion by 30%
−4	Reduce infusion by 75%
−5	Hold infusion

interventions, for example, moving patients into the prone position. The type, combination and dose of agent used (Table 12.4) influence the risk of increased side effects. Propofol is one of the most common sedation drugs used in critical care. Propofol is a short-acting medication that results in a decreased level of consciousness and lack of memory for events. Side effects include apnoea,

TABLE 12.4 Commonly used sedation drugs in adult critical care [9].

Medication	Example infusion composition	Concentration	Central access	Peripheral access
Propofol	1% 2%	10 mg/mL 20 mg/mL	✓	✓
Midazolam	50 mg in 50 mL 100 mg in 50 mL	1 mg/mL 2 mg/mL	✓	✓
Clonidine	750 µg in 50 mL	15 µg/mL	✓	✓

hypotension, and nausea and vomiting. Midazolam may be used instead of propofol if the patient has cardiovascular instability; however, there is the risk of drug accumulation and delirium. Clonidine is an additional sedative agent that can be considered for use in patients difficult to sedate. Side effects may include hypotension, bradycardia and a negative chronotrope effect; therefore caution should be used in patients with low cardiac output or impaired ventricular function [10].

It should also be noted that drugs may become unavailable or supplies may be limited. In addition, infusion/syringe pumps to administer medications may become limited, affecting how sedation and analgesia are provided. Therefore because sedation regimens may need to vary, it is essential that staff have a good working knowledge of commonly used medications, their side effects and access to protocols and guidelines for administration. COVID-19 patients with a tracheostomy are typically managed with reduced or no sedation. In a pandemic setting, this may have several advantages, including the need for less intensive nursing care, as the patient may be able to assist with rolling or moving. Fewer pumps will be needed at the bedside, which may be advantageous if there is a shortage of drugs or devices. Care may be overseen by non-critical care staff who are not experienced in managing continuous infusions of sedation and analgesia [11].

Neuromuscular blockade

Patients requiring neuromuscular blocking agents must be deeply sedated (i.e., RASS −4 or −5); this should be achieved prior to starting any neuromuscular blocking agents. Deep sedation is recommended to reduce the risk of the patient becoming aware. Sedation infusions should not be weaned when neuromuscular agents are in progress. Train-of-four monitoring and clinical assessment should be routinely used to monitor the depth of the neuromuscular blocking agent and to confirm that all drug-related actions or effects have ceased.

TABLE 12.5 Commonly used neuromuscular blocking agents used in critical care [9].

Medication	Example infusion composition	Concentration	Central access	Peripheral access
Atracurium	250 mg in 25 mL 500 mg in 50 mL	10 mg/mL	✓	X
Cisatracurium	150 mg in 30 mL	5 mg/mL	✓	X
Rocuronium	500 mg in 50 mL	10 mg/mL	✓	X

In critical care, neuromuscular blocking agents are used to reduce patient–ventilator asynchrony, maintain oxygenation and monitor lung-protective ventilation strategies and prone position. Bolus drugs may be used to assess the patient's response before starting an intravenous infusion. Commonly used drugs include rocuronium and pancuronium. Commonly used continuous infusions of neuromuscular agents include cisatracurium and atracurium (Table 12.5). In the event of an accidental extubation, patients receiving a neuromuscular agent will not be able to breathe spontaneously; therefore immediate access to emergency airway equipment, including a bag and valve mask, must be positioned at the patient's bedside [12].

Pain assessment

Most patients in critical care will experience pain. Pain may be caused when undertaking routine critical care, for example, turning, endotracheal suctioning, nursing and medical procedures or wound care. Untreated pain leads to impaired mobility, prolonged ventilation, psychological stress and possible delirium. Conscious patients should be encouraged to self-report when assessing pain using validated scoring tools such as the Numerical Rating Scale 0–10 scale, with 0 being no pain and 10 being the worse pain imaginable. However, ventilated patients may not be able to communicate due to the endotracheal tube or use of sedation. Reliance on vital signs to assess pain has been found to be ineffective and a poor judge regarding severity of pain. It is recognized that changes in vital signs may indicate the presence of pain or discomfort, and these therefore must be regarded as a prompt for nurses to complete a pain assessment. The Critical Care Pain Observation Tool is an approved and validated tool to assess pain (Table 12.6) [4].

Causes of pain include fear, helplessness, loss of control due to the condition that led to hospitalization/critical care admission and/or the unfamiliar critical care environment itself. Loss of memory and time due to the type and amount of

TABLE 12.6 Critical Care Pain Observation Tool [13].

Indicator	Description	Score
Facial expression	Non-muscular tension observed	Relaxed, natural 0
	Presence of frowning, brow lowering, orbit tightening, levator contraction	Tense 1
	All the foregoing facial movements plus eyelid tightly closed	Grimacing 2
Body movements	Does not move at all (does not necessarily mean absence of pain)	Absence of movements 0
	Slow, cautious movements, touching or rubbing the pain site, seeking attention through movements	Protection 1
	Pulling tube, attempting to sit up, moving limbs/thrashing, not following commands, striking at staff, trying to climb out of bed	Restless 2
Muscle tension	No resistance to passive movements	Relaxed 0
	Resistance to passive movements	Tense, rigid 1
	Strong resistance to passive movements, inability to complete them	Very tense or rigid 2
Compliance with the ventilator (intubated patients) Or vocalization (extubated patients)	Alarms not activated, easy ventilation Alarms stop spontaneously	Tolerating ventilator or movement 0
	Asynchrony, blocking ventilation, alarms frequently activated	Coughing but tolerating 1 Fighting ventilator 2
	Talking in normal tone or no sound Sighting, moaning Crying out, sobbing	Talking in normal tone or no sound 0 Sighting, moaning 1 Crying out, sobbing 2
Total range 0–8		

drugs administered. Medication and/or condition may prevent communication and/or limit understanding of their current situation. Background noises, for example, alarms, phones ringing, may contribute to an inability to sleep. There may also be frustration at not being able to do things for themselves or feel they are not getting better. Other sensations include thirst, hunger, hot, cold, cramps, nausea, itching and boredom. As a consequence, pain management involves consideration of both pharmacological and non-pharmacological approaches.

Non-pharmacological approaches

Non-pharmacological approaches include speaking with the patient, always using their name, explaining procedures before starting (even if they are not

TABLE 12.7 Commonly used pain medication concentrations used in adult critical care [9].

Medication	Example infusion composition	Concentration	Central access	Peripheral access
Morphine	50 mg in 50 mL 100 mg in 50 mL	1 mg/mL 2 mg/mL	✓	✓
Fentanyl	2.5 mg in 50 mL	50 µg/mL	✓	✓
Alfentanil	25 mg in 50 mL	500 µg/mL	✓	✓
Remifentanil	2 mg in 40 mL 5 mg in 50 mL	50 µg/mL 100 µg/mL	✓ ✓	✓ ✓

conscious) and providing reassurance. Include the patient in all activities where possible and check whether or not they are in pain. Distraction therapies, for example, music, may be helpful and every effort should be made to establish and maintain care routines. Fundamental nursing care includes position changes, mouth care to prevent thirst and maintain oral hygiene, checking if the patient is warm or cold, checking whether the patient is hungry, use of therapeutic touch to provide comfort and reassurance, appropriate use of alarm settings and reduction of additional sources of discomfort such as bright lights.

Pharmacological approaches

Pharmacological approaches include use of validated pain assessment tools, proactive use of analgesia prior to nursing or medical interventions, for example, prior to dressing changes, position changes, use of 'as required' ('pro re nata') analgesia for breakthrough pain and inclusion of pain assessment as part of the daily multidisciplinary ward round.

Common continuous opioid analgesia infusions used include fentanyl, alfentanil, remifentanil and morphine (Table 12.7). Opioid infusions may impair gut mobility, leading to intolerance to feeding, constipation and malnutrition. Abdominal distention may impair ventilation and lead to nausea and vomiting, increasing the risk of aspiration [1].

Delirium

Delirium, previously termed 'ICU syndrome' or 'ICU psychosis', is a common clinical syndrome characterized by disturbed consciousness, cognitive function or perception, which has an acute onset and fluctuating course. It usually develops over 1–2 days. It is a serious condition that is associated with poor outcomes [14]. Delirium can be hypoactive or hyperactive; however, it can be mixed in some people.

ICU-induced delirium has been found not to resolve spontaneously and as a consequence may last several weeks or months. The risk of delirium in mechanically ventilated patients increases for each day the patient remains sedated and/or immobilized. Delirium is triggered by the use of antianxiety medications, age, environment (busy, noisy, brightly lit units), sleep disruption caused by scheduled monitoring and nursing care, for example, taking vital signs, bloods and turning. To identify possible causes of delirium, the pneumonic THINK is used [15]:

- T: Toxic situations (heart failure, shock, dehydration, organ failure and drugs).
- H: Hypoxaemia.
- I: Infection, sepsis or immobilization.
- N: Non-pharmacological interventions used (eyeglasses, hearing aids, reorientation, sleep protocols and noise control).
- K: K+ (potassium) or other electrolyte problems.

Risk factors associated with delirium include dementia, history of hypertension and history of alcoholism or critical illness at time of admission [4]. The Confusion Assessment Method for ICU (CAM-ICU) is a reliable and valid screening tool to assess patients for delirium [4]. It has been specifically designed for use in critical care settings and has a high level of sensitivity when compared to the American Psychiatric Association criteria for delirium [16]. The CAM-ICU tool is widely used internationally.

Patients with COVID-19 who have been admitted to critical care are at risk of delirium due to several factors, including direct central nervous system (CNS) invasion, CNS inflammatory mediators release, secondary effects from multiorgan failure, effects of sedative strategies, prolonged mechanical ventilation, immobilization and environmental factors, including social isolation and limited interaction with family [17] (Fig. 12.1). In many countries, families have been prevented from visiting relatives in hospital to reduce the risk of transmission. However, this poses challenges for nurses, with communication to families and patient's next of kin only possible via telephone. In response to this, the use of technology such as iPads has been introduced to allow patients, relatives and staff to communicate more effectively [18].

To reduce the impact of critical illness and outcomes, the ABCDEF bundle is an organizational model with evidence-based interventions [19]. The bundle allows for improved communication amongst the critical care team, standardization of care and reduction of the risk of delirium and weakness (Table 12.8).

Medications such as haloperidol (1–2 mg) may be indicated; however, it has to be noted that haloperidol only reduces the associated agitation and/or aggression, not the duration of delirium.

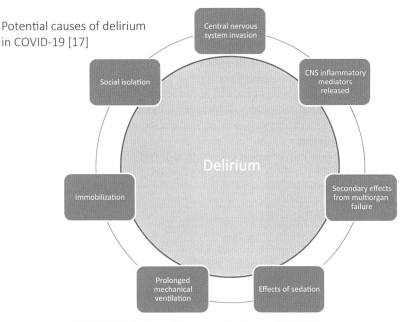

Potential causes of delirium
in COVID-19 [17]

FIGURE 12.1   Potential causes of delirium in COVID-19.

TABLE 12.8 ABCDEF bundle [19].

A	Assess for and manage pain
B	Perform: • Spontaneous Awakening Trial – daily interruption in sedation drugs • Spontaneous Breathing Trial – daily trial of spontaneous breathing as appropriate
C	Choice of sedation and analgesia
D	Delirium monitoring and management
E	Early mobility
F	Family engagement

Conclusion

This chapter has explored the importance of the inclusion of neurological assessment in the care of COVID-19 patients in critical care. It is accepted that both analgesia and sedation are integral elements of critical care patient pathways. The challenge for critical care nurses is that patients may not be able to indicate the presence of pain or distress and discomfort. Every effort must therefore be made to proactively monitor and assess patients through the use of validated assessment tools. Delirium is yet another challenge for the critical care nurse. With little or no prior knowledge of the patient it may be hard to recognize early signs indicating the onset of delirium. As cited earlier, there are validated tools and models suitable for use in critical care, and these should be used routinely to prevent or reduce the onset of delirium.

Neurological care is complex and multifaceted. This area of care in terms of COVID-19 is still in its infancy. However, as evidence continues to grow, it is demonstrated that not only is it an issue in the acute phase of the illness but there is a legacy effect that can continue after the period of critical illness. It is therefore essential that nurses make every effort to protect patients and recognize potential problems early to minimize the possibility of long-term neurological problems.

References

[1] Hanidziar D, Bittner EA. Sedation of mechanically ventilated COVID-19 patients: challenges and special considerations. Anesth Analg 2020;131(1):e40–1. https://doi.org/10.1213/ANE.0000000000004887.

[2] Helms J, et al. Neurologic features in severe SARS-CoV-2 infection. Letter to the editor. N Engl J Med April 15 2013;20. ePub.

[3] Jevon P. Neurological assessment: part 2 pupillary assessment. Nurs Times 2008;104(28):26–7.

[4] Garrett KM. Best practices for managing pain, sedation and delirium in the mechanically ventilated patient. Crit Care Nurs Clin 2016;28:437–50.

[5] Berkow L, Kanowitz A. COVID-19 putting patients at risk of unplanned extubation and airway providers at increased risk of contamination. Anaesth Analgesia 2020;131(1):e41–3. https://doi.org/10.1213/ANE.0000000000004890.

[6] Hruska P. Early mobilization of mechanically ventilated patients. Crit Care Nurs Clin 2016;28:413–24. North America.

[7] ICU Delirium. Richmond Agitation-Sedation Scale (RASS). 2018. Available at: www.icudelirium.org/docs/RASS.pdf.

[8] Intensive Care Foundation. Handbook of mechanical ventilation – a user's guide. 2015. [London].

[9] Intensive Care Society. Medication concentrations in adult critical care areas. 2017. London www.ics.ac.uk.

[10] Intensive Care Society. Review of best practice for analgesia and sedation in the critical care. 2014. [London].

[11] National Tracheostomy Safety Project. Advice for patients with a tracheostomy in the Coronavirus pandemic. 2020. [UK] www.tracheostomy.org.

[12] Intensive Care Society. Critical care guidance relating to the Tier 3 Alert of supplies of Atracurium, Cisatracurium and Rocuronium. 2020. https://icmanaesthesiacovid-19.org/news/critical-care-guidance-relating-to-the-tier-3-alert-of-supplies-of-atracurium-cisatracurium-and-rocuronium.

[13] Gelinas C, Fillion L, Puntillo KA, et al. Validation of the critical-care pain observation tool in adult patients. Am J Crit Care 2006;15(4):420–7.

[14] National Institute for Health and Care Excellence. Delirium: prevention, diagnosis and management. Clin Guidel (CG) 2019;103. https://www.nice.org.uk/guidance/cg103/chapter/introduction.

[15] National Institute for Health and Care Excellence. THINK delirium in intensive care. 2020. https://www.nice.org.uk/sharedlearning/think-delirium-in-intensive-care.

[16] Gusmao-Flores D, FigueiraSalluh JI, Chalhub RA, et al. The confusion assessment method for the intensive care unit (CAM-ICU) and intensive care delirium screening checklist (ICDSC) for the diagnosis diagnosis of delirium: a systematic review and meta-analysis of clinical studies. Crit Care 2012;16:R115.

[17] Kotfis K, Williams Roberson S, Wilson JE, Dabrowski W, Pun BT, Ely EW. COVID-19: ICU delirium management during SARS-CoV-2 pandemic. Crit Care 2020;24(1):176. https://doi.org/10.1186/s13054-020-02882-x. Published 2020 Apr 28.

[18] Massachusets General Hospital. Virtual Care connects patients and families during COVID-19 pandemic. 2020. https://www.massgeneral.org/news/coronavirus/virtual-care-connects-patients-and-families.

[19] Marra A, Ely EW, Pandharipande PP, Patel MB. The ABCDEF bundle in critical care. Crit Care Clin 2017;33(2):225–43. https://doi.org/10.1016/j.ccc.2016.12.005.

Chapter 13

Resuscitation in COVID-19

Daniel Paschoud, Chris Carter, Joy Notter

Chapter Outline

Introduction

Resuscitation is arguably one of the most physically and mentally challenging tasks that a healthcare professional can undertake. Patients admitted due to COVID-19 have an increased propensity for rapidly progressive respiratory failure, necessitating critical care admission [1], and it is essential that early consideration should be made for advanced care planning. It is important to establish with the patient and the people that are important to them what treatments are likely to be of benefit. This includes discussing the implications of critical care admission and resuscitative treatment. Therefore, this chapter focuses on the impact of the additional stressors and challenges that must be considered when delivering resuscitative treatment during the COVID-19 pandemic. It reviews the evidence and guidance that has been developed to help healthcare professionals carry out resuscitation for patients in the presence of the clinical symptoms of COVID-19. It also explains practical application of the guidance developed in the context of usual and expanded critical care environments. Before carrying out resuscitation, there are some important factors that all teams need to be aware of, as they may vary according to the clinical environment. As many ward and specialist settings have been reconfigured or expanded due to the pandemic, carrying out in situ simulation of cardiac arrests can be of benefit

COVID-19: A Critical Care Textbook. https://doi.org/10.1016/B978-0-7020-8383-9.00013-0

to teams. These enable staff to practice and familiarize themselves with the non-technical skills and equipment unique to this situation and through this can contribute to improving patient outcomes [2]. Teams can check all staff are aware of where level 3 personal protective equipment (PPE) is kept, who the team leader will be if there is a cardiac arrest, what other team roles need to be assigned, and how the cardiac arrest team is summoned. Information can be shared regarding where the cardiac arrest equipment is kept and its layout. Should any members not know how to use the equipment (e.g., defibrillator), appropriate training can be given before an actual clinical incident arises. During the pandemic the redeployment of staff has made need for retraining much more frequent, and it is recommended that skills assessments are made when staff move to a new, and possibly very different, clinical environment.

It is a cause for concern that in some settings contradictory advice has been given. For example, in the UK, both the International Liaison Committee on Resuscitation and Resuscitation Council (UK) [3,4] identify cardiopulmonary resuscitation (CPR) as an aerosol-generating procedure (AGP), yet this was not reflected in Public Health England guidance which deemed CPR not to be an AGP [5]. As a result, at a local level, hospitals have implemented and adapted their own specific algorithms, for example, all inpatients are considered COVID-19 suspected regardless of reason for admission [6]. In consequence, healthcare teams must have clear communication regarding actions for a cardiac arrest in a ward setting.

Advanced care planning

Advanced care planning is key to efficient care delivery, therefore nurses need to know the documentation used and understand the legal and clinical implications of the decisions made. A Do Not Attempt Cardiopulmonary Resuscitation (DNA-CPR) order is a legal document. However, some clinicians and the general public have a perception that this also dictates the level of treatment that a patient receives, seeing it as the clinical equivalence of 'giving up' [7], which is not true. While it does specify that CPR (cardiopulmonary resuscitation) will not be initiated if a patient does suffer cardiac arrest, it does not dictate the 'ceilings of care' for the patient, or dictate whether the patient should be admitted to critical care. The setting and timing of the discussions needed for advanced care planning should also be carefully considered [8]. There are legal considerations to the discussion of DNA-CPR orders. To prevent misunderstandings and miscommunication the BMA, RCN and RC (UK) have all sought to clarify the current legal and ethical considerations of this process through the publication of a joint statement [9]. Nursing professional organizations have also published further guidance emphasizing the need for an individualized, patient-centred approach to this process during the current pandemic [10].

Treatment escalation plans are becoming more commonplace in acute healthcare settings. These set out clearly for members of the multidisciplinary team what interventions the clinical team, in discussion with the patient/next of kin, has decided would be appropriate should the patient deteriorate. This may include whether the patient should be admitted to critical care or receive non-invasive ventilation (NIV). These plans are beneficial if they are made prior to deterioration as they provide the opportunity for the patient and their next of kin to ask questions and to have the risks/benefits and rationale of the decisions being made explained to them. This can also be an opportunity for practitioners to discuss the current prognosis and expected clinical course. To support clear documentation of all aspects of decisions made, several organizations have collaborated to form the ReSPECT process [11], which provides resources to support these conversations and a standardized format of documentation to accompany the shared discussions.

Professional and patient safety

The International Liaison Committee on Resuscitation (ILCOR) states that chest compressions have the potential to generate aerosols and recommends that healthcare professionals should wear appropriate PPE for resuscitation attempts [4]. The aerosol-generating procedures (AGPs) essential to advanced life support (ALS) represent a hazard of contamination and infection to anyone in the immediate vicinity as droplets are expelled from the patient into the area around them. In some clinical areas, such as critical care, where the nature of care services provided means there are already AGPs ongoing, team members may already be wearing the appropriate PPE for resuscitation. This should lead to reducing the delay in commencing chest compressions.

It has to be accepted that, in this current pandemic, there are situations where the team may not be wearing full PPE, and consequentially will not be in an appropriate state of preparedness to immediately start chest compressions. Therefore, to minimize delays, in areas where there is a possibility of sudden presentation of possible or confirmed COVID-19 cases, such as the emergency department, full PPE should be readily available and accessible, with all practitioners aware of its location.

After a cardiac arrest has been recognized, during the COVID-19 pandemic there needs to be a careful balance between risks versus benefit. It is essential to ensure that there are sufficient team members with an appropriate skill-mix for the attempt, whilst minimizing exposure to AGPs by restricting staff in the environment to those essential for the resuscitation attempt [2]. RC (UK) also advises placing a simple oxygen mask on the patient's face, to limit the dispersal of contaminated droplets [2]. During resuscitation attempts this may pose an increased risk of transmission of COVID-19 to responders and other patients within the vicinity [12]. This is an important consideration, because previous infectious disease outbreaks have shown the transmission of viruses to healthcare professional despite them wearing PPE during resuscitation attempts [13,14].

Recognition of the deteriorating patient

Individuals with severe COVID-19 disease may develop respiratory failure without accompanying circulatory failure. They can deteriorate rapidly, with the unique feature of requiring a sudden increase in oxygen requirements without significant changes to other parameters and symptoms of respiratory distress. Early warning scoring tools may not be sensitive enough to detect such changes [15]. In consequence, this may impact on recognition of the deteriorating patient and the team response to clinical deterioration.

The decision to initiate resuscitation during a pandemic is complex. In some settings it has been proposed that CPR should not be initiated without adequate PPE [16]. In the early phase of the UK pandemic, reports of restrictive resuscitation practices include the recommendation that patients in cardiac arrest outside the emergency department can only be given defibrillator treatment if they have a 'shockable' rhythm [17]. While these practices have been condemned as they do not follow national or international guidance, nevertheless they will have impacted on patient survival rates. Therefore, hospitals must have appropriate plans in place for the management of the deteriorating patient for all cardiac arrest situations.

Recognition of cardiac arrest

Prior to the COVID-19 pandemic, a 'Look, Listen, Feel' detection method was advised [18], whereby the practitioner would bring their face close to the patient's mouth to recognize cardiac arrest. In the presence or possibility of COVID-19, this method has considerable potential for contamination and/or infection of the practitioner. In consequence, the guidelines have been updated, and now recommend that the practitioner still performs the look, listen and feel detection, but stands further distanced from the patient's face [2] and for no longer than 10 s. If the patient's breathing is absent or abnormal (agonal gasping), then chest compressions should be initiated.

Manual pulse palpation at the carotid can be performed if you have been trained to do so. However, there is now some documented evidence of false positives/negatives arising during manual pulse palpation [19]. Therefore, if the practitioner has not been trained in this technique, confirmation of cardiac arrest should be specified as above by solely checking for 'normal breathing'.

Calling for help

Activation of the cardiac arrest team should be the first consideration after confirmation of a cardiac arrest. The process for this can differ as it tends to be based on local guidelines. Clinical areas such as critical care or the emergency department may manage cardiac arrests 'internally', whilst most ward environments will call for the cardiac arrest team via a telephone/

bleep system. All staff need to be fully orientated to local guidelines and all communication should make it clear when and if there is a potential risk of COVID-19 infection.

Assessment of rhythm

Consideration should be made for early application of an automated external defibrillator (AED) or manual defibrillator to determine the patient's cardiac arrest rhythm. Previously, chest compressions would have been immediately initiated after confirmation of cardiac arrest, but the change in approach has been made because this intervention is thought to produce additional aerosolized droplets, increasing the potential for contamination and/or disease transmission. The benefit of a 'defibrillator-first' approach is that it can be carried out whilst other team members don PPE and prepare to provide chest compressions. Once the defibrillation pads are applied to the patient, rhythm assessment can take place.

Today, many in-hospital defibrillators have an AED mode. This enables the machine to automatically detect the cardiac rhythm of the patient and recommend the appropriate treatment strategy (shockable or non-shockable). When using the AED mode, it is important to follow all cues the machine provides to ensure correct rhythm analysis, as continuing CPR during this process can in some instances lead to inappropriate treatment. The risk/benefit of using the defibrillator in the AED mode is complex. It is possible that the AED mode can decrease the time to the first defibrillation attempt [12]. However, there is an argument that using the manual mode can decrease 'preshock pauses' and in doing so can theoretically improve the chances of achieving return of spontaneous circulation (ROSC) [13]. Nevertheless, those that have only been trained to use the AED mode should avoid the use of the manual mode. This requires additional training, as it needs rapid identification of cardiac arrest rhythms, and a good understanding of the safe defibrillation sequence.

Throughout ALS the cardiac arrest rhythm is reassessed every 2 minutes and treatment administered as per the appropriate branch of the algorithm. As previously highlighted; chest compressions generate ECG artefacts that can lead to misinterpretation of the cardiac arrest rhythm. Therefore, CPR needs to be paused to enable effective analysis of the rhythm to be made. As with any interruption in chest compressions, this pause should be minimized and take no longer than 5 seconds [20]. If the defibrillator is being used in manual mode, then the team leader should have a good view of the defibrillator screen prior to pausing CPR.

There are four classifications of cardiac arrest rhythm. The Resuscitation Council (UK) [RC (UK)] has produced guidance and an algorithm to maximize the effectiveness for resuscitation in the context of COVID-19 [2] (Fig. 13.1). The management of these is separated into two branches of the algorithm – shockable and non-shockable.

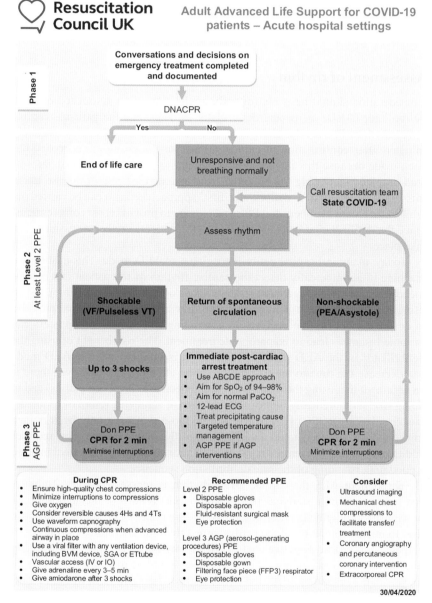

FIGURE 13.1   Advanced life support for COVID-19 patients in an acute hospital setting. *[Reproduced with the kind permission of the Resuscitation Council (UK).]*

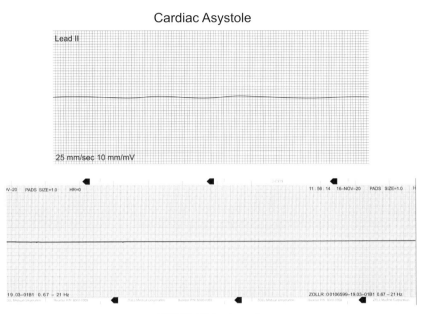

FIGURE 13.2   Asystole.

Non-shockable rhythms

Non-shockable rhythms include pulseless electrical activity (PEA) and asystole. PEA is a rhythm that would be compatible with life, and therefore a member of the team should attempt to palpate a carotid pulse if this is seen (Fig. 13.2). If there is insufficient cardiac output to generate a pulse, CPR should be recommenced. Asystole can be characterized as a 'flat' line, although typically there may be some small amounts of drift. It is indicative of an absence of mechanical and electrical cardiac activity. Once a non-shockable rhythm has been identified, CPR should be immediately reinitiated.

Shockable rhythms

Cardiac arrest rhythms which can be restored by defibrillation include pulseless ventricular tachycardia (pVT) and ventricular fibrillation (VF). pVT is characterized as a tachycardia, with regular broad QRS complexes (Fig. 13.3A). VF can be recognized as a disorganized irregular rhythm, with no discernible P, Q, R, S, or T waves (Fig. 13.3B). This is due to random twitching and electrical activity across the muscle fibres of the heart.

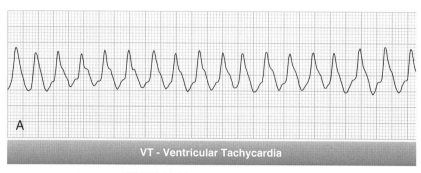

FIGURE 13.3A   Ventricular tachycardia.

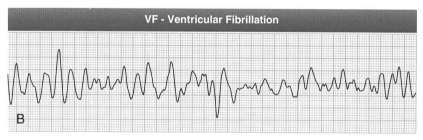

FIGURE 13.3B   Ventricular fibrillation.

Defibrillation

If the patient is in a shockable rhythm, early defibrillation is associated with a greater likelihood of ROSC [21]. RC (UK) recommends that whilst the defibrillator is charging, CPR is recommenced with all other team members (other than the CPR provider) instructed to stand clear. Once the defibrillator is charged the CPR provider should also be instructed to stand clear, the shock administered, and CPR immediately recommenced [18]. If, as per the modified COVID-19 algorithm, the defibrillator has been attached prior to CPR and the patient is in a shockable rhythm, up to three shocks can be administered in an attempt to convert the patient to a rhythm compatible with life whilst awaiting others to commence chest compressions.

It is vital that safety is maintained throughout any defibrillation attempt. Due attention must be paid to the area within which the shock is being administered. No-one should be in contact with the patient or their immediate area, this prevents any risk of shock transference, which could potentially harm team members.

There are some concerns around the perceived risk of ignition caused by defibrillation due to the presence of oxygen. The European Resuscitation Council (ERC) reports that there is no evidence of this occurring when self-adhesive pads were used. The ERC advises that practitioners exercise caution when performing defibrillation, ensuring that direct sources of oxygen such as a mask or nasal cannula be removed to 1 metre away from the patient, and also that a ventilation bag should remain attached to an ETT or SGA during shock delivery [20]. In critical care, patients may be ventilated during CPR to prevent disconnection of the ventilator, a mandatory mode of ventilation with a set respiratory rate of 12 breaths per minute and an FiO_2 of 1.0 can be set. If disconnection from the ventilator is required, the ventilator should be placed into the stand-by mode, to prevent aerosolization of particles. During defibrillation, the charge should be delivered during expiration to prevent transthoracic impedance.

Chest compressions

Chest compressions should be delivered at a rate of 100–120 compressions per minute, vertically to a depth of 5–6 cm (or a third of the anterior–posterior depth of the patient's chest). Chest compressions should be delivered with the heel of the practitioner's hand in the centre of the low half of the patient's sternum [22]. Since the onset of the pandemic, patients with severe COVID-19 who are unstable have been observed to deteriorate, resulting in cardiac arrest while in the prone position, as this has been increasingly used to improve oxygenation for both intubated and conscious patients with COVID-19 [23,24]. Returning a patient to the supine position is the optimum for resuscitation. However, as this necessitates a coordinated team procedure, particularly for a patient who is intubated, it may not be immediately possible. In consequence, CPR can be commenced in the prone position. The Intensive Care Society has highlighted that there is limited evidence available regarding this, but recommends a two-handed technique between the scapula [25]. The ERC also endorses this technique, recommending a similar rate and depth as supine (usual) CPR [26]. It has to be noted that applying sternal counter-pressure may help to generate higher mean arterial pressures (MAPs) [27].

Consistent quality of chest compressions is positively associated with ROSC [28]; however, provision of effective chest compressions is physically tiring, and in this pandemic providers are also encumbered by PPE and thus are likely to tire sooner. As the provider tires there will be a drop off in the overall quality of chest compressions. Swapping providers often to maintain efficacy of chest compressions is an easy means of negating this. Therefore, team members need to monitor the quality of chest compressions. This can be achieved visually, using a metronome or using CPR feedback devices where available, or a diminishing $EtCO_2$ trace can be another indicator of compression provider fatigue. In COVID-19 areas, the number of responders may be limited due to the availability of staff and those who are wearing appropriate CPR. In consequence, teams may need to swap providers more frequently and rotate all team members (excluding the team leader) to perform CPR.

Throughout the resuscitation attempt any interruption in CPR should be no greater than 5 s. This is due to the rapid drop-off in perfusion pressure when there is no CPR. In order to minimize the interruption when swapping CPR providers, it should be clearly established and stated as to who will be taking over, and a clear countdown should be given "3…2…1". To further minimize interruptions in CPR these changeovers should, where possible, be integrated with the necessary pauses for rhythm assessment [20].

In some settings mechanical chest compression devices may be available. These devices perform chest compressions at a set rate, which is particularly useful for prolonged cardiac arrests where team member fatigue becomes a significant risk to chest compression quality. It is important to recognize that as with all medical equipment, these devices require specific training to ensure they are applied appropriately and effectively. In addition, in the COVID-19 environment, equipment may not be immediately available and after the resuscitation attempt will need to be appropriately decontaminated.

Vascular access

If the patient has an existing intravenous (IV) access this should be assessed for patency. If this is insufficient or not patent, further access should be gained to enable the administration of drugs and fluids. The peripheral IV cannula is the equipment most healthcare professionals will be familiar with, so inserting a wide-bore cannula bilaterally may be the most readily available means to gain IV access, however, in the absence of cardiac output the patient's vasculature will peripherally shut down, making this more challenging.

Intraosseous (IO) access is a good alternative to traditional vascular access with equipment available in many in-hospital environments. The correct insertion technique for these devices requires additional training, however there are several benefits to using IO during cardiac arrest. For a trained practitioner, the land-marking and insertion process can be faster than typical central venous catheter (CVC) placement [29]. Evidence has shown that medications can take as little as 3 s to reach the heart via the humeral head intraosseous route, demonstrating its viability for resuscitative purposes [30]. However, there are several contraindications to intraosseous access, including the presence of any hardware/trauma in the limb and recent attempted/successful previous IO insertion.

CVC or central lines are typically established in critical care patients. It is important to account for the additional dead space in these lines, therefore, flushing with an appropriate volume of 0.9% sodium chloride is required so that the entire dose is administered.

Drugs

During cardiac arrest it may be appropriate to administer drugs, depending on the rhythm, timing and cause of the cardiac arrest. Adrenaline (epinephrine) (1 mg)

[31] has been given historically in cardiac arrest due to its alpha-adrenergic vaso-constrictive effects which increase cerebral and coronary perfusion [20]. It is administered in both the shockable and non-shockable algorithm but is dependent on the initial cardiac arrest rhythm [20]. In non-shockable rhythm, adrenaline (epinephrine) is administered immediately, and subsequent doses should continue to be administered every 3–5 min. Practically speaking, this would be after every alternate rhythm assessment, at 4-min intervals.

If the initial rhythm is shockable, then this adrenaline regime should only be initiated after the third shock has been administered. If the patient converts to a non-shockable rhythm, then the adrenaline regime is commenced. Once the adrenaline regime has commenced it continues irrespective of subsequent cardiac arrest rhythms.

Amiodarone is an antiarrhythmic drug that slows atrioventricular conduction and appears to improve the response to defibrillation [20]. It is administered if the patient is in a shockable rhythm, this should be administered after the third shock [32]. After a fifth shock a further dose of 150 mg should be considered [20]. There are ongoing clinical studies for both medications and their impact on cardiac arrest outcomes and guidelines may be updated in the future dependent on the quality and significance of evidence.

Airway management

Placement of an advanced airway allows for continuous (asynchronous) chest compressions. This should be done by a practitioner who is experienced and competent in airway management. Ideally, the patient will be intubated using an endotracheal tube (ETT), however a supraglottic airway (SGA), such as an iGel or LMA, may be used. To minimize the risk of exposure to team members a viral filter should be integrated into the airway circuit [26]. Once the airway is secured the patient's ventilation will need to be continuously monitored to ensure adequate oxygenation. This can be done in three ways: by visually confirming bilateral chest movement, by auscultation of the chest to confirm bilateral air entry and via end-tidal CO_2 ($EtCO_2$) monitoring. However, in COVID-19 it may not be possible to auscultate the chest due to PPE and the risk of breaching PPE. In consequence, other methods may be relied upon. $EtCO_2$ waveform monitoring also has other applications for cardiac arrest management. Interpreting the values and waveforms generated during the resuscitation attempt can be indicative of quality of CPR, prognostication and ROSC [33–35].

Reversible causes and aetiology

As management of the cardiac arrest proceeds from basic to ALS, any potentially reversible causes of the cardiac arrest should be considered and addressed. These are often described as the four 'H's and 'T's [20]. 'H's include hypoxia, hypovolaemia, hypo/hyperkalaemia (including metabolic disorders) and hypothermia. 'T's include tension pneumothorax, tamponade, toxins and thrombosis. The aim of resuscitation is to restore spontaneous circulation as soon as possible, therefore those factors most likely to be contributing to the cardiac arrest should be addressed first. Key to this process is understanding the potential aetiology of cardiac arrest in the context of COVID-19. In the presence of COVID-19 infection hypoxaemia secondary to acute respiratory distress syndrome (ARDS) is a potential causative factor of cardiac arrest. Consequentially, an early consideration should be made to ensure hypoxia is effectively and definitively countered with advanced airway management, and manually ventilated with a high concentration of oxygen [26].

There is some evidence to suggest COVID-19 severity is associated with electrolyte imbalance, specifically sodium, potassium and calcium deficiencies [36]. There is also growing evidence of acute kidney injury in COVID-19 patients requiring renal replacement therapy (RRT) [37]. Significant electrolyte derangement is associated with increased risk of sudden cardiac arrest [38]. As a constituent of effective cardiac arrest management, electrolytes should be checked using a rapid point-of-care test, typically an arterial blood gas (ABG) sample, to detect any electrolyte imbalance. This should then be corrected appropriately.

The evidence of increased risk of acute kidney injury in COVID-19 patients [31] has been partially attributed to hypovolaemia, secondary to fever and dehydration common in this patient group [39]. This can be corrected intra-arrest with crystalloid intravenous fluids such as 0.9% sodium chloride or Hartmann's solution in boluses [20].

Hypothermia is unlikely in the context of in-hospital COVID-19 patients but should be ruled out for patients arriving as out-of-hospital cardiac arrests (OHCAs). This can be corrected with warmed IV fluid infusion and external warm air [38].

Emerging evidence has suggested there has been an increased incidence of thromboembolic events in COVID-19 patients [40]. In the context of cardiac arrest, the treatment for this is fibrinolytic drugs. Once fibrinolytic drugs have been administered resuscitation may continue for 60–90 min in order to ensure that this medication can break down any potential thrombus [38].

COVID-19 patients are often intubated due to ARDS and consequentially can have poor lung compliance when they undergo sustained periods of ventilation. These are known risk factors for pneumothorax formation [41]. A multicentre case series has also demonstrated that these patients are more prone to pneumothoraces [42]. A pneumothorax can be detected by observing the chest for asymmetrical chest movement and auscultating for asymmetrical poor or absent air entry. If there is an ETT in situ, then unintentional endobronchial intubation is a possible differential diagnosis. Tracheal deviation is another indication of tension pneumothorax; however, this is a late sign, therefore the team should not wait to observe this prior to initiating treatment. The initial treatment for a tension pneumothorax is a needle thoracentesis (decompression). Historically this would be performed using a wide-bore cannula in the second intercostal space, midclavicular line. There is now evidence to suggest that performing this in the fifth intercostal space on the mid-axillary line has a higher success rate [43]. A tension pneumothorax must be definitively treated by inserting an underwater sealed chest drain or by thoracostomy [38].

Cardiac tamponade can be difficult to detect intra-arrest and will likely only be present with an indicative history such as chest trauma or recent cardiac surgery. Use of ultrasound intra-arrest can be used to diagnose this, however it should only be attempted by trained clinicians to avoid prolonged interruption to chest compressions [20]. If this is detected then a resuscitative thoracotomy would be indicated.

Where there is evidence of toxic or therapeutic substances contributing to the cardiac arrest, expert help via online databases or poison centres should be sought to administer the appropriate antidote where possible [38]. Prolonged resuscitation may be required if this may enable the excretion or metabolization of a causative toxin or for an antidote to take effect [38].

Communication

Co-ordination of the multidisciplinary team during a cardiac arrest is pivotal to ensuring that interventions are enacted promptly as the situation develops. The use of PPE will impact the identification of team members and communication. A popular means of overcoming this has been to write names/roles in large lettering on the front of PPE, being mindful to not compromise these protective barriers. As team members will be wearing PPE this will lead to vocal muffling and the loss of lip-reading ability and other non-verbal facial communication cues. Teams should be aware of this negative factor and be mindful of unnecessary noise and the flow of communication during the resuscitation attempt. Use of closed-loop communication has been demonstrated to improve this [44]. Establishing and using gestures and other non-verbal communication tools with colleagues may also be helpful.

Termination of attempt

As the situation develops and after potentially reversible causes of the cardiac arrest have been addressed, the team should consider the potential success of this resuscitation attempt. The ERC states that *"Asystole for more than 20 min during ALS in the absence of a reversible cause is generally accepted as an indication to abandon further resuscitation attempts. However, there are reports of exceptional cases that do not support the general rule, and each case must be assessed individually"* [45]. The termination of a resuscitation attempt can be challenging. The decision ultimately rests with the team leader, however there may be a benefit to asking others involved in the resuscitation attempt if they have any concerns/treatments to suggest prior to discontinuing [43].

The evidence gathering related to in-hospital cardiac arrest outcomes for COVID-19 patients is ongoing. Current studies have demonstrated outcomes for COVID-19-positive cardiac arrest cases range from 13.2% to 42% ROSC rate [46,47], with one study in Wuhan, China, reporting a 2.9% survival at 30 days [46]. However, a case series in the United States reported no patients survived to hospital discharge [47].

Post-resuscitative care

If the patient shows any signs of life/a pulse, then post-resuscitative care should begin. As soon as ROSC is confirmed the team around the patient should then co-ordinate assessment using an airway, breathing, circulation, disability and exposure (A,B,C,D,E) systematic approach. The airway is assessed to ascertain if the patient is tolerating any airway interventions and whether they are still effective. If this is an SGA or ETT this can be confirmed by the same means as set out above. Sedation and analgesia infusions may need to be initiated in order for the airway device to be tolerated. In COVID-19 areas it may not be possible to confirm air entry. However, an ABG should be taken to confirm effective gas exchange and detect any respiratory failure. Determining SpO_2 using a peripheral sensor may not be immediately possible due to the patient's poor perfusion state. In the critical care environment consider if the patient can now be connected to a ventilator and further optimized. It is advisable to perform a chest X-ray as part of post-resuscitative care to detect any potential chest resuscitation-related injury such as a pneumothorax and confirm the placement of any medical devices such as an ETT [48].

Post-cardiac arrest, patients may be cardiovascularly unstable. Therefore, patients should be assessed to confirm that the patient does not require further intervention due to cardiac arrhythmias in order to prevent rearrest. If the patient is unstable then it may be of benefit for one member of the team to maintain a position palpating the carotid pulse, in case the patient deteriorates into a PEA, as cardiac monitoring would continue to show a rhythm compatible with life in this case. A 12-lead ECG should be taken, in order to detect cardiac arrhythmias, heart blocks or myocardial ischemia that may have contributed to the cardiac arrest.

A neurological assessment of the patient should take place to assess the patient post-arrest. This should include a Glasgow Coma Scale score and pupillary reflexes. More advanced neurological assessment including imaging may be required and contribute to prognostication [49].

The ERC advises the avoidance of hyperthermia in the post-arrest period, which can be common in the first 48 h [49]. This can be achieved via several methods including active cooling pads and antipyretics. There is additionally ongoing evidence gathering around the process of targeted temperature management (TTM) and the optimal maintenance temperature that may positively impact neurological recovery post-ROSC [49].

Equipment

All surfaces and equipment involved in the cardiac arrest should be decontaminated or disposed of appropriately and as per manufacturer guidance, particularly those associated with airway management [50]. PPE should be carefully removed to avoid contamination.

Debriefing

There are often practical learning points to be taken away from a resuscitation attempt. Sharing these as a team after the event gives an opportunity to highlight any concerns they have, or anything they thought went well and should be replicated. This can contribute to improved patient outcomes [51]. There are various models that have been developed for debriefing. A debriefing can be as simple as thanking team members for their work and asking if they have any immediate questions or concerns about the event. The level of sudden deterioration and mortality during the pandemic is of a scale unseen by many healthcare professionals. Team members may feel that they benefit psychologically from debriefing [52]. Acute healthcare settings should ensure that anyone exposed to a resuscitative event has access to psychological support.

Conclusion

There are several alterations to typical resuscitation practice that healthcare professionals should be aware of as they deliver care during the pandemic. Effective dissemination of these adjustments alongside preparation of teams and environments will benefit resuscitation attempts. The causative factors of cardiac arrest in COVID-19 and the outcomes for these patients are the topic of ongoing research, and so there is a need for practitioners to continuously update themselves, enabling them to provide evidence-based practice to this vulnerable patient group.

References

[1] World Health Organization. Clinical management of severe acute respiratory infection (SARI) when COVID-19 disease is suspected. https://www.who.int/docs/default-source/coronaviruse/clinical-management-of-novel-cov.pdf

[2] Resuscitation Council (UK). Statements on COVID-19: in-hospital settings. Resuscitation Council UK. www.resus.org.uk/covid-19-resources/statements-covid-19-hospital-settings

[3] Couper K, Taylor-Phillips S, Grove A, Freeman K, Osokogu O, Court R. COVID-19 in cardiac arrest and infection risk to rescuers: a systematic review. Resuscitation 2020;151:59–66.

[4] Perkins GD, Morley PT, Nolan JP, et al. International Liaison Committee on Resuscitation: COVID-19 consensus on science, treatment recommendations and task force insights. Resuscitation 2020;151:145–7. https://doi.org/10.1016/j.resuscitation.2020.04.035.

[5] Public Health England. Guidance COVID-19 personal protective equipment (PPE). 2020. www.gov.uk/government/publications/wuhan-novel-coronavirus-infection-prevention-and-control/covid-19-personal-protective-equipment-ppe#ppe-guidance-by-healthcare-context.

[6] Thorne CJ, Ainsworth M. COVID-19 resuscitation guidelines: a blanket rule for everyone? Resuscitation 2020;153:218.

[7] Gibbs AJO, Malyon AC, Fritz ZBMC. Themes and variations: an exploratory international investigation into resuscitation decision-making. Resuscitation 2016;103:75–81.

[8] Hall CC, Lugton J, Spiller JA, Carduff E. CPR decision-making conversations in the UK: an integrative review. BMJ Support Palliat Care 2020;9:1–11.

[9] Resuscitation Council UK. Guidance from the British Medical Association, the Resuscitation Council (UK) and the Royal College of Nursing. 2016.

[10] Royal College of Nursing. COVID-19 guidance on DNACPR recommendations and verification of death. 2020. [London].

[11] Resuscitation Council UK. ReSPECT for healthcare professionals. Resuscitation Council UK; 2020. www.resus.org.uk/respect/respect-healthcare-professionals.

[12] Crook P. Cardiopulmonary resuscitation in the COVID-19 era - will the risk-benefit shift in resource-poor settings? Resuscitation 2020;151:118.

[13] Christian MD, Loutfy M, McDonald LC, et al. Possible SARS coronavirus transmission during cardiopulmonary resuscitation. Emerg Infect Dis 2004;10:28793.

[14] Nam H-S, Yeon M-Y, Park JW, Hong J-Y, Son JW. Healthcare worker infected with Middle East Respiratory Syndrome during cardiopulmonary resuscitation in Korea, 2015. Epidemiol Health 2017;39:12.

[15] Pimentel MAF, Redfern OC, Hatchb R, Young DJ, Tarassenko L, Watkinson P. Trajectories of vital signs in patients with COVID-19. Resuscitation 2020;156:99–106.

[16] Kapoor I, Prabhakar H, Mahajan C. Cardiopulmonary resuscitation in COVID-19 patients – to do or not to? J Clin Anaesth 2020;65:109879.

[17] Mahase E, Kmietowicz Z. Covid-19: doctors are told not to perform CPR on patients in cardiac arrest. BMJ 2020;368. https://doi.org/10.1136/bmj.m1282.

[18] Resuscitation Council UK. Guidelines: in-hospital resuscitation. 2015. www.resus.org.uk/library/2015-resuscitation-guidelines/hospital-resuscitation.

[19] Tibballs J, Russell P. Reliability of pulse palpation by healthcare personnel to diagnose paediatric cardiac arrest. Resuscitation 2009;80(1):61–4.

[20] Soar J, Nolan JP, Böttiger BW, Perkins GD, Lott C, Carli P, et al. European resuscitation Council guidelines for resuscitation 2015: section 3. Adult advanced life support. Resuscitation 2015;95:100–47.

[21] Chan PS, Krumholz HM, Nichol G, Nallamothu BK. Delayed time to defibrillation after in-hospital cardiac arrest. N Engl J Med 2008;358:9–17.

[22] Perkins GD, Handley AJ, Koster RW, Castrén M, Smyth MA, Olasveengen T, et al. European Resuscitation Council guidelines for resuscitation 2015: section 2. Adult basic life support and automated external defibrillation. Resuscitation 2015;95:81–99.

[23] Munshi L, delSorbo L, Adhikari NKJ, Hodgson CL, Wunsch H, Meade MO, et al. Prone position for acute respiratory distress syndrome: a systematic review and meta-analysis. Ann Am Thoracic Soc 2017;14:S280–8.

[24] Elharrar X, Trigui Y, Dols AM, Touchon F, Martinez S, Prud'Homme E, et al. Use of prone positioning in nonintubated patients with COVID-19 and hypoxemic acute respiratory failure. J Am Med Assoc 2020;323:2336–8.

[25] Intensive Care Society. Prone position guidance in adult critical care [internet]. 2019. www.ics.ac.uk/ICS/ICS/Pdfs/Prone_Position_Guidance_in_Adult_Critical_Care.aspx.

[26] European Resuscitation Council. European resuscitation Council COVID-19 guidelines. 2020.

[27] Mazer SP, Weisfeldt M, Bai D, Cardinale C, Arora R, Ma C, et al. Reverse CPR: a pilot study of CPR in the prone position. Resuscitation 2003;57(3):279–85.

[28] Wallace SK, Abella BS, Becker LB. Quantifying the effect of cardiopulmonary resuscitation quality on cardiac arrest outcome: a systematic review and meta-analysis. Circulation 2013;6(2):148-56.

[29] Leidel BA, Kirchhoff C, Bogner V, Stegmaier J, Mutschler W, Kanz K-G, et al. Is the intraosseous access route fast and efficacious compared to conventional central venous catheterization in adult patients under resuscitation in the emergency department? A prospective observational pilot study. Patient Saf Surg 2009;6(2):148–56.

[30] Montez DF, Puga T, Miller L, Saussy J, Davlantes C, Kim S, et al. 133 intraosseous infusions from the proximal humerus reach the heart in less than 3 seconds in human volunteers. Ann Emerg Med 2015;66(4):S47.

[31] British National Formulary. Adrenaline/epinephrine. 2020. https://bnf.nice.org.uk/drug/adrenalineepinephrine.html.

[32] British National Formulary. Amiodarone hydrochloride. 2020. https://bnf.nice.org.uk/drug/amiodarone-hydrochloride.html#interactions.

[33] Sheak KR, Wiebe DJ, Leary M, Babaeizadeh S, Yuen TC, Zive D, et al. Quantitative relationship between end-tidal carbon dioxide and CPR quality during both in-hospital and out-of-hospital cardiac arrest. Resuscitation 2015;89:149–54.

[34] Paiva EF, Paxton JH, O'Neil BJ. The use of end-tidal carbon dioxide ($EtCO_2$) measurement to guide management of cardiac arrest: a systematic review. Resuscitation 2018;123:1–7.

[35] Lui CT, Poon KM, Tsui KL. Abrupt rise of end tidal carbon dioxide level was a specific but non-sensitive marker of return of spontaneous circulation in patient with out-of-hospital cardiac arrest. Resuscitation 2016;104:53–8.

[36] Lippi G, South AM, Henry BM. Electrolyte imbalances in patients with severe coronavirus disease 2019 (COVID-19). Ann Clin Biochem 2019;57(3):262–5.

[37] Ronco C, Reis T, Husain-Syed F. Management of acute kidney injury in patients with COVID-19. Lancet Respirat Med 2020;8:738–42.

[38] Truhlář A, Deakin CD, Soar J, Eldin G, Khalifa A, Alfonzo A, et al. European resuscitation council guidelines for resuscitation 2015: section 4. Cardiac arrest in special circumstances. Resuscitation 2015;95:148–201.

[39] Selby NM, Forni LG, Laing CM, Horne KL, Evans RDR, Lucas BJ, et al. Covid-19 and acute kidney injury in hospital: summary of NICE guidelines. BMJ 2020;369. www.nice.org.uk/guidance/.

[40] Marginean A, Masic D, Brailovsky Y, Fareed J, Darki A. Difficulties of managing sub massive and massive pulmonary embolism in the era of COVID-19. J Am Coll Cardiol 2020;2(9):1383–7.

[41] Rankine JJ, Thomas AN, Fluechter D. Diagnosis of pneumothorax in critically ill adults postgraduate. Med J 2000;76:399–404.

[42] Martinelli AW, Ingle T, Newman J, Nadeem I, Jackson K, Lane ND, et al. COVID-19 and pneumothorax: a multicentre retrospective case series. Eur Respir J 2020;56(5):2002697.

[43] Laan D, Vu TDN, Thiels CA, Pandian TK, Schiller HJ, Murad MH, et al. Chest wall thickness and decompression failure: a systematic review and meta-analysis comparing anatomic locations in needle thoracostomy. Injury 2016;47(4):797–804.

[44] El-Shafy IA, Delgado J, Akerman M, Bullaro F, Christopherson NAM, Prince JM. Closed-loop communication improves task completion in paediatric trauma resuscitation. J Surg Educ 2018;75(1):58–64.

[45] Bossaert LL, Perkins GD, Askitopoulou H, Raffay VI, Greif R, Haywood KL, et al. European resuscitation council guidelines for resuscitation 2015. Section 11. The ethics of resuscitation and end-of-life decisions. Resuscitation 2015;95:302–11.

[46] Shao F, Xu S, Ma X. In-hospital cardiac arrest outcomes among patients with COVID-19 pneumonia in Wuhan, China. Resuscitation 2020;155:18–23.

[47] Sheth V, Chishti I, Rothman A, Redlener M, Liang J, Pan D. Outcomes of in-hospital cardiac arrest in patients with COVID-19 in New York city. Resuscitation 2020;155:3–5.

[48] Resuscitation Council (UK). Guidelines: post-resuscitation care. 2015. [London].

[49] Nolan JP, Soar J, Cariou A, Cronberg T, Moulaert VRM, Deakin CD, et al. European resuscitation council and European society of intensive care medicine guidelines for post-resuscitation care 2015. Section 5 of the European resuscitation council guidelines for resuscitation 2015. Resuscitation 2015;95:202–22.

[50] Resuscitation Council (UK). Resuscitation Council UK Statement on COVID-19 in relation to CPR and resuscitation in acute hospital settings. 2020. [London].

[51] Edelson DP, Litzinger B, Arora V, Walsh D, Kim S, Lauderdale DS, et al. Improving in-hospital cardiac arrest process and outcomes with performance debriefing. Arch Intern Med 2008;168(10):1063–9.

[52] Gilmartin S, Martin L, Kenny S, Callanan I, Salter N. Promoting hot debriefing in an emergency department. BMJ Open Qual 2020;9(3):e000913.

Chapter 14

Care of the critically ill obstetric patient

Alice Sadra, Chris Carter, Joy Notter

Chapter Outline

Introduction

Maternal critical care is an area less discussed than other parts of obstetric, midwifery and critical care practice [1]. High-income countries have relatively few pregnancies complicated by severe illness and, in consequence, midwives and critical care teams in these areas may well have limited opportunities to develop and practice the specialized expertise required to care for the critically ill peripartum woman [2]. However, in low-resource settings, maternal admissions are suggested to be between 0.13% and 4.6%, with high mortality [3]. Studies have identified that critical care nurses often have concerns regarding competence and confidence in caring for obstetric patients [4,5]. In addition, midwifery education programmes do not always contain rigorous acute nursing care competencies, leading to anxiety for midwives when caring for acutely ill or deteriorating patients [6]. Therefore, this chapter has been designed to provide an overview of critical care nursing and midwifery issues that need to be considered in the care of critically ill suspected or confirmed COVID-19 obstetric patients.

COVID-19

The COVID-19 pandemic is a rapidly emerging and evolving situation. Research into therapies and treatments are continuously advancing but there remains limited understanding of the impact of COVID-19 infection in mothers and their babies [7]. Pregnant women, without underlying co-morbidities known to increase the risk of contracting the virus, are not thought to be more susceptible to COVID-19 than the general population [8]. However, as Favre et al. [9] point out, changes to the immune system during pregnancy may mean that pregnant women are more vulnerable to severe illness once infected with COVID-19 and therefore, as a precautionary measure, most countries have identified pregnant women as being clinically vulnerable in order to reduce the risk of transmission and potential complications [10]. This is corroborated by the UK Obstetric Surveillance System (UKOSS) [11], a research platform that gathers national data about specific severe complications of pregnancy. In a 2-month prospective observational cohort study a total of 427 pregnant women, most of whom were in their final trimester were admitted to hospital with confirmed COVID-19, 41 received Level 3 care, four required extracorporeal membrane oxygenation (ECMO) at a tertiary centre and five died. A total of 262 women gave birth or experienced a pregnancy loss while admitted [6], with severe illness appearing to be more common in later pregnancy. This UKOSS study highlighted a disproportionate amount of women from Black and minority ethnic groups admitted to hospital in pregnancy with COVID-19. A finding supported by Khalil et al. [12] in a systematic review and analysis of 86 studies into COVID-19 infection and pregnancy.

Physiological changes during pregnancy

Pregnancy is divided into three trimesters with the management of maternal critical illness being dependent on what stage the pregnancy is at. The first trimester is between weeks 1 and 12, the second is from weeks 13 to 26 and the third is from week 27 until delivery. In pregnancy, major and continued physical adaptations occur in maternal physiology [12]. Admitting an unwell pregnant woman presents challenges for the critical care interdisciplinary team with regard to their altered physiology, the unborn baby and in terms of how COVID-19 affects pregnancy [13]. Consequently, a team approach to care is essential to maintain the unique needs of the maternal patient in critical care. It has to be noted that given the limited evidence and information on the critical care management of a pregnant women with suspected or confirmed COVID-19, the principles of care may be guided by the same guidelines as for non-pregnant patients [14]. Therefore, it is important for critical care nurses to understand and recognize the normal altered physiological functions of pregnancy.

Safety considerations

Any patient with suspected or confirmed COVID-19 must be cared for by staff wearing personal protective equipment (PPE) in accordance with local and national infection control guidelines. In addition, midwifery and obstetric staff attending to a pregnant woman with COVID-19 must be aware of the potential modes of transmission to other women and the strategies needed to prevent this. These include the need for appropriate fit testing of a FFP3 mask together with donning and doffing training for PPE (Chapter 4).

Patient assessment

As with all critical care patients, the seriously ill pregnant patient requires the comprehensive monitoring and recording of observations. Assessment should include a review of the woman's past medical and obstetric history in order that deviations from the individual patient's baseline are recognized. Patient assessment should follow the ABCDE approach (Chapter 6). It is important to note that the patient must be holistically assessed, as different professionals may focus on different aspects, for example, the midwives may focus on foetal heart rate, observing for bleeding or assessing uterine contractions [13]. However, to maintain a structured situational awareness (Chapter 3), a systematic approach to assessment should be followed. Where a modified early obstetric warning system (MEOWS) track and trigger system is used, the aim is to identify serious illness amongst pregnancy women early, taking account of the altered physiology. However, it has to be noted there are no standardized MEOWS, and these tools compliment holistic assessment of the deteriorating patient [14].

Airway

In a self-ventilating woman with suspected or confirmed COVID-19, supplementary oxygen should be given to keep oxygen saturations >95% unless otherwise directed. The risk of the pregnant COVID-19 patient developing respiratory failure is high for several reasons. If the patient is in the third trimester or it is a multiple pregnancy then there may be difficulty in positioning the patient to optimize lung expansion. Hypoxia can occur due to altered lung function, diaphragmatic splitting by the large uterus and increased oxygen consumption. In addition, reduced gastric motility and relaxation of the lower oesophageal sphincter increases the risk of aspiration.

Emergency endotracheal intubation is considered a high-risk procedure in all situations, with Lapinsky [16] warning that up to 40% of patients may have significant hypoxic or hypotensive episodes. Therefore, in some situations, it may be appropriate to use non-invasive ventilation (NIV) (Chapter 7) to prevent or delay the need for intubation. However, as Mazlan [17] points out, using NIV is associated with increased risks of gastric aspiration, and therefore, it may only be appropriate in women who are fully conscious and able to maintain their own airway. It is important to note that fluid shift and generalized vasodilation caused during pregnancy may increase the possibility of laryngeal oedema, making airway assessment difficult and increasing the risk of a challenging intubation [14]. In addition, the physiological changes of pregnancy may result in rapid hypoxia during any period of hypoventilation [1].

As outlined in Chapter 8, presumed and confirmed COVID-19 patients requiring mechanical ventilation may be assessed and treated by dedicated teams. These teams have the specialist skills to intubate patients in emergency departments and ward areas then, once the airway is secured, transferring them to the critical care unit. Preparatory communication is essential, and the specialist team must liaise with the critical care doctors and nurse-in-charge, so that the smooth transfer, admission to critical care and ongoing care needs can be facilitated.

Intubation is an aerosol-generating procedure. Therefore, appropriate PPE must be worn and a team trained in airway management is essential. In some settings, intubation checklists [18] may be used to maintain safety. During any intubation a plan for escalation in the event of failure to intubate should also be made [18]. Immediate access to difficult airway equipment is essential, ideally together with a video laryngoscope. In addition to the risk of laryngeal oedema, a difficult airway is more likely in pregnancy due to poor positioning, obesity and large or engorged breasts. A smaller endotracheal tube may be necessary, because of the increased airway vascularity, however, the size of the tube will be assessed by the practitioner performing the intubation [19]. During intubation there is an increased risk of pulmonary aspiration of gastric contents, which is especially significant during pregnancy. Early tracheal intubation decreases this risk and, as advocated by Schnettler et al. [20], a rapid sequence induction (RSI) should be routinely used. In some situations, it may be appropriate to administer an H2 antagonist or antacid [1].

Post-intubation interventions include continuous capnography monitoring and a chest X-ray to check the position of the ETT. Chest imaging should not be delayed because of concerns of possible maternal and foetal exposure to radiation, as maternal well-being is paramount [21]. The use of lead shielding to the abdomen may be used to mitigate any risk to the baby [22].

Breathing

As pregnancy progresses, there is an increased metabolic and oxygen demand, leading to greater maternal respiratory effort. In addition, many women experience a degree of dyspnoea throughout pregnancy due to the expanding uterus and pregnancy-induced hyperventilation [23]. As Soma-Pillay et al. [24] point out, it is considered normal for a pregnant woman to have a mild, fully compensated respiratory alkalosis. However, acidosis may be seen in critical illness due to decreased buffering capacity [14]. Additionally, pregnant women will typically have a larger tidal volume of between 150 and 200 mL, leading to a minute volume increase of 40% compared to non-pregnant women of a similar age [14].

Severe COVID-19 causes a viral pneumonia, which can lead to acute respiratory failure and organ dysfunction. Liu et al. [25] suggest that the physiological adaptations found in pregnancy, such as increased oxygen demand and an altered immune system, may increase a woman's susceptibility to respiratory pathogens. In consequence, the changes to respiratory physiology may result in pregnant women being less tolerant to hypoxia [26]. It is important to recognize that although dyspnoea may be seen in the context of a healthy pregnancy, failure to identify the signs of respiratory deterioration can result in delays in escalation of treatment. Changes in respiratory rate, pattern and depth are useful indicators of deterioration due to respiratory, metabolic, cardiovascular or neurological conditions [14]. It is important to note that young, otherwise healthy women have efficient compensatory mechanisms and are capable of maintaining normal oxygen saturations but may abruptly deteriorate and decompensate [21]. Therefore, extra vigilance in this vulnerable group for signs of deterioration is crucial.

Due to the changes in respiratory physiology, invasive ventilation (Chapter 8) may be more difficult and should be overseen and directed by the critical care team. Direct care must be provided by appropriately experienced nursing and medical staff, who have the expertise to manage and adjust ventilator settings, depending on the patient's clinical status and arterial blood gases. Chest physiotherapy is crucial in all ventilated patients, especially those admitted with respiratory conditions. It is essential that the physiotherapy team is made aware that the patient is pregnant.

In patients who develop severe acute respiratory distress syndrome (ARDS), it is technically challenging to place a pregnant woman in the prone position, particularly in the second or third trimesters. There is little evidence regarding the effectiveness and use of prone positioning in pregnant women [26], as pregnancy is often considered to be a contraindication to prone position. However, there is some emerging evidence to support the use of the prone position in pregnancy [14,27]. Indeed, Hirshberg et al. [15] point out that the prone position may be considered an option if other strategies aimed at improving gas exchange have failed and describe the prone position of a COVID-19 patient who was successfully proned at 28-weeks pregnant. Data on the use of ECMO in the pregnant patient with COVID-19 are limited. However, it has been used as a rescue therapy for pregnant patients with H1N1 influenza and should be considered in the case of severe refractory respiratory failure in COVID-19 [28].

Circulation

In many settings, pregnant women will carry with them their medical notes, which may well include baseline data of vital signs and blood results. These can be used as a reference guide when assessing health status and planning care. Haemodynamic changes are a part of the normal physiological response to pregnancy and these include increased volume expansion and vasodilation in response to increased tissue metabolic demand [13,29,30]. In addition to this, physiological anaemia may result in reduced oxygen-carrying capacity, consequently, the monitoring of haemoglobin levels and oxygen saturation levels are essential.

Cardiac output changes throughout the pregnancy: by 8 weeks gestation, cardiac output has increased by 20%, and at 24 weeks cardiac output is estimated to have increased by up to 45% [23,29]. Blood pressure drops approximately 10 mmHg by the second trimester, despite a gain in intravascular volume of 30%–50% [30]. Decreased systemic vascular resistance occurs due to the effects of progesterone causing generalized vasodilation [13]. Simultaneously, the maternal heart rate increases by 15–20 beats per minute throughout pregnancy [13]. As a consequence, these physiological changes, together with other compensatory mechanisms, may potentially conceal the more commonly recognized and expected features of shock.

Positioning of the patient can affect the haemodynamic status of women. From 20 weeks of pregnancy onwards, the supine position can cause uterine compression of the vena cava to such an extent that cardiac output may fall by as much as 30%–40%, this is termed 'supine hypotension' [13]. This can rapidly lead to maternal collapse, which can often be resolved by turning the patient into the left lateral position [31]. Alternatively, left manual displacement of the uterus may be performed. This is a simple manoeuvre using an "up, off and over" technique, whereby the uterus is lifted up and away from the right side of the patient and over to the left [31]. Both the left lateral position and manual displacement of the uterus aim to relieve the pressure on the inferior vena cava.

Emerging evidence from the COVID-19 pandemic indicates that the virus is associated with cardiovascular pathologies including myocarditis, myocardial infarction, dysrhythmias and venous thromboembolism (VTE) [32]. It is recommended that echocardiograms should be performed in pregnant patients with severe COVID-19 to assess cardiac function [32]. It has to be noted that pregnancy is a hypercoagulable state, with women being more likely to develop a deep vein thrombosis (DVT) or pulmonary embolism (PE). This is thought to be a protective strategy that reduces the risk of haemorrhage during birth or miscarriage [13]. However, in high-income countries, due to other risk factors including obesity, smoking and maternal age greater than 35, DVTs are linked to high mortality and morbidity, with PEs being a leading case of maternal death [31]. As outlined in Chapter 6, critically ill COVID-19 patients are at high risk of developing VTE [33]. Assessment of the calves for signs of swelling and inflammation should be undertaken to observe and monitor for signs of VTE. VTE prophylaxis includes graduated compression stockings and all pregnant women admitted with confirmed or suspected COVID-19 should receive prophylactic low-molecular-weight heparin (LMWH) unless birth is expected within 12 h [21]. If there are any concerns regarding the possibility of a PE then pulmonary angiography should be considered and the use of treatment-dose LMWH or a heparin infusion discussed with senior critical care and obstetric doctors together with specialist pharmacists [21].

Disability (neurological) care

Acute neurological events are rare in women of childbearing age [34], but it is important to point out that where there is uncontrolled pregnancy-induced hypertension, it can lead to an increased risk of seizure and cerebrovascular accidents (CVAs) [14,34]. Confusion, anxiety and reduced level of consciousness may be caused by hypotension and/or hypoxia. It is therefore essential that a comprehensive neurological assessment using the Glasgow Coma Scale and checking of pupillary reflexes (Chapter 12) should be included as part of the assessment. In addition, blood glucose levels should be assessed for hypo- or hyperglycaemia.

A ventilated obstetric patient will require sedation and opiate infusions in order to facilitate ventilation and manage pain and distress (Chapter 12). Pelayo et al. [35] describe the successful care of a third-trimester patient with severe COVID-19 who required the additional use of neuromuscular blockade in order to achieve adequate ventilation. As with all drugs administered on the critical care unit, careful consideration must be given when prescribing for the obstetric patient. Sedation scoring must be followed as per department policy and it is the critical care nurses' responsibility to titrate sedative drugs so that issues of under- and over-sedation are avoided [13].

Renal

Pregnancy has a widespread effect on renal physiology, affecting virtually all aspects of kidney function [36]. The kidneys increase in size with glomerular filtration rate (GFR) rising early to a peak between 40% and 50% higher than measured prepregnancy, resulting in decreased levels of urea and creatinine [14]. Antidiuretic hormone (ADH) production is suppressed, resulting in altered urine output and increased thirst, which in turn leads to a reduction in osmolality and consequently lower serum sodium levels. Concurrently, rising levels of progesterone protect the mother from hypokalaemia [36]. Urinary tract infections (UTIs) are more common in pregnant women due to the changes in immunity and altered urinary tract physiology predisposing the woman to infection [14].

Current evidence indicates that COVID-19 may have serious implications for the kidneys and renal function, affecting an estimated 20%–40% of patients admitted to critical care [37]. It is important to note that patients who develop an acute kidney injury (Chapter 11) are more likely to require escalation to critical care with a higher likelihood of being ventilated, which is associated with a higher mortality [38]. Data on the use of renal replacement therapy (RRT) in critically ill, COVID-19 obstetric patients are limited. However, in the event of an obstetric patient requiring RRT, insertion of intravenous lines (VasCaths) will most likely be in the internal jugular or subclavian veins, both to reduce the risk of infection and because pressure from the gravid uterus may impede the blood flow through femoral lines to the haemofilter. The use of anticoagulation to maintain the RRT filter circuit should follow the usual policies and guidelines, with input from critical care and obstetric consultants together with senior specialist pharmacists.

Gastrointestinal and metabolic

Effects on the gastrointestinal tract and metabolism during pregnancy are caused primarily by hormonal changes, specifically the effects of progesterone, and are not solely limited to the physical consequences of the gravid uterus [13]. Common issues experienced by pregnant women include nausea, vomiting and heartburn. Hyperemesis gravidarum (HG), which affects 0.3%–3.6% of pregnant women [39], is diagnosed when there is severe, protracted nausea and vomiting, together with more than 5% prepregnancy weight loss, dehydration and electrolyte imbalance [40]. This can result in hospital treatment for rehydration and electrolyte replacement. The growing uterus displaces the stomach and increases pressure in the stomach, potentially causing gastro-oesophageal reflux and increasing the risk of aspiration. This is a key concern when caring for a pregnant patient who requires invasive or non-invasive ventilation.

Malnutrition in critical illness is an enduring issue worldwide [41], with the provision of adequate, appropriate nutrition in critical care having a strong correlation with reduced length of ventilator dependence, improved outcome, fewer hospital-acquired infections and decreased length of hospital admission [42]. Early enteral feeding is a common intervention in critical care, however, specialist dietician input must be sought to provide appropriate energy requirements based on co-morbidities and current pathology [42]. As pregnancy results in reduced oesophageal tone and slower gastric emptying [14] there is the potential for increasing the risk of pulmonary aspiration of stomach contents during enteral feeding. Critical care nurses must be aware of this when initiating enteral feeding, repositioning or suctioning the pregnant patient. The position of a nasogastric tube should be checked and confirmed before it is used for feed or drug administration. Prokinetic drugs can be used to improve gastrointestinal motility and it is recommended that gut-protective medications should be administered routinely to reduce the risk of aspiration [43].

Immune system

The maternal immune system adapts and changes to maintain a careful equilibrium between protecting the growing foetus from immunologic attack without disrupting protection against infection [44]. Sepsis in pregnancy remains a major cause of maternal death within both high- and low-income countries [21]. As outlined in Chapter 1, COVID-19 is a viral infection with growing evidence that sepsis and associated multiorgan dysfunction can be a serious complication [45]. As identified by Bridwell et al. [46], the normal haemodynamic changes of pregnancy – vasodilation, tachycardia and increased cardiac output – may mask the signs of sepsis, leading to the potential for its under-recognition. It is essential that the critical care nurse caring for the obstetric patient is aware of this altered physiology in order for early recognition of deterioration and to allow for prompt escalation to senior staff. Careful attention to infection control guidelines, aseptic techniques with invasive lines and monitoring together with routine surveillance swabs and culturing need to be adhered to. Most patients in critical care will have at least daily blood tests sent, which allows for early identification of elevated inflammatory and infection markers.

Maternal cardiac arrest

Maternal arrest is an incredibly challenging scenario and there is the high likelihood that most members of the critical care and responding teams will have had little experience of it. In the event of a pregnant patient on the critical care unit suffering a cardiac arrest, resuscitation should follow the same local and national resuscitation guidelines as used in all adult patients [1] (see Chapter 13). A maternal and neonatal cardiac arrest call should be put out via the emergency number to the hospital's switchboard as expert obstetric and paediatric support may be required.

If the patient is 20 or more weeks pregnant, left manual displacement of the uterus should be performed. This is a simple manoeuvre using an "up, off and over" technique whereby the uterus is lifted up and away from the right side of the patient and over to the left [32]. Historically, the woman was tilted to the left to facilitate more effective cardiopulmonary resuscitation (CPR), however displacing the uterus manually is more efficient, simpler to facilitate and allows for easier access to the chest and airway [47]. If the patient is in a shockable rhythm then defibrillation should occur without delay with the defibrillator pads being applied in the same way as for any patient in cardiac arrest [47]. At the same time as effective CPR is being carried out, the potential cause(s) of the cardiac arrest need to be considered and treated.

In the event of no return of spontaneous circulation (ROSC) within 4 min and the woman is 20 weeks pregnant or over, a perimortem caesarean section should be undertaken [47]. This is the emergency surgical delivery of the baby and is a procedure primarily aimed at aiding maternal resuscitation rather than saving the life of the foetus [47]. The purpose of delivering the baby and placenta is to improve venous return and cardiac output together with reducing oxygen demand for more effective CPR [32,47].

An in-hospital perimortem caesarean section will be performed in situ, with the patient not being transferred to the operating theatre as this would lead to unnecessary delay. As the patient is already in cardiac arrest there will be minimal blood loss and no anaesthetic is required. The only immediate equipment that is required is a scalpel [32,47]. However, the massive obstetric haemorrhage protocol should still be initiated, in case of significant bleeding [40]. If resuscitation is successful then definitive management of the surgical wound and ongoing critical care will take place. It is recommended that if a critically ill >20-week pregnant woman is admitted to critical care, a clear plan for performing a perimortem caesarean section should be made [40,47].

Care of the post-partum COVID-19-confirmed patient in critical care

Rationales for post-partum care will depend on the severity of COVID-19 infection, whether or not the woman is ventilated and the mode of birth. Following caesarean section the patient will have an abdominal wound and potentially a subcutaneous drain [48]. The majority of critical care nurses have experience of looking after surgical patients including women post-caesarean section. Postoperative nursing care during the pandemic should broadly follow the same strategies regarding airborne infection control precautions and the pathophysiology of COVID-19. If the patient has had a vaginal birth there is the possibility of a perineal wound or damage requiring sutures or even packing. This, together with the assessment of lochia, the bloody vaginal discharge occurring after birth, will require midwifery and obstetric input [14]. Pain may be an issue following either caesarean or vaginal birth. Regular pain scoring should be performed and analgesia administered as prescribed or required. The patient should be reviewed by the critical care team with the obstetric team if her pain is not well managed or increasing.

A confirmed COVID-19 diagnosis does not preclude breastfeeding, indeed mothers with the virus are being encouraged to breastfeed their babies [27]. However, if the mother requires critical care in a COVID-19 area, the baby would not be able to be brought to the mother due to concerns regarding infection control. If the mother has capacity, discussions regarding the expressing of colostrum and breast milk can be had, ideally led by or with support from the midwifery and neonatal feeding team.

Psychological care

Obstetric critical care admission is almost invariably an unanticipated event and one that is undoubtedly terrifying for the woman and her family. This is obviously exacerbated with regard to COVID-19 by fears due to the pandemic and because of visiting restrictions in many hospitals. International studies of women's experiences of maternal critical care have highlighted common themes of fear, disempowerment and shock during the emergency itself, coupled with potential long-term psychological and emotional effects including flashbacks [49].

In the awake post-partum woman in the critical care unit, the implications of separation from her baby must be addressed. Prior to the pandemic, it may have been possible for the baby to be brought to the critical care unit, however, due to COVID-19 infection controls this is unlikely to be allowed. In addition, visitors, including the partner, may not be allowed. Staff wearing PPE and the highly charged critical care environment are hugely stressful. Strategies to improve the situation include allowing pictures of her baby and family at the bedside and the use of an iPad or mobile phone to video call family members for virtual visiting of the baby and mother. The kindness and empathy of staff to support maternal bonding cannot be overestimated in this situation.

In the sad event of a neonatal death, most hospital labour wards have access to a cold cot, which allows bereaved parents to spend time with their stillborn baby [50]. This must be an option for awake mothers in critical care if the situation arises, even in the context of the pandemic. The mother, and indeed the critical care staff, will need to be supported by specialist midwives. If the mother is sedated and ventilated and therefore potentially unaware that her baby has died, close liaison with midwifery and obstetric staff regarding bereavement support when appropriate is crucial.

Teamwork

Caring for a critically ill maternal patient with suspected or confirmed COVID-19 is an incredibly challenging scenario; staff must have access to support and support mechanisms such as clinical supervision. It is accepted that effective maternal care is delivered by teams rather than individuals [14]. Indeed, failure between professionals and at handover has been associated with detrimental patient care [51]. COVID-19 restrictions may prevent the presence of midwives and obstetricians working in critical care, due to the risk of infecting others, therefore, communication and visits by these members of the team may be limited or conducted via telephone. As indicated above, the majority of critical care nurses may have limited experience in caring for critically ill obstetric patients and it is vital to escalate concerns, no matter how trivial they may seem. To improve communication during an emergency situation, tools such as the SBAR or RSVP may be used (Table 14.1).

Conclusion and recommendations

Successful care of critically ill pregnant or post-partum patients necessitates a multidisciplinary team approach with daily input from obstetricians and midwives being crucial to provide early recognition of deterioration and guidance of specialist care [2]. Critical care units must have policies and guidelines for the admission and care of pregnant women. During the COVID-19 pandemic

TABLE 14.1 Communication tools [14].

General points to consider when calling for help:
- Know who to call, e.g., nurse in charge, critical care resident, obstetric registrar.
- If 'bleeping' or 'paging' stay by the phone to respond to the call-back.
- Confirm who you are speaking to.
- Have the patient's medical notes/records and vital signs available.
- Use a structured approach to handover as outlined below.
- If you are not happy with the response, escalate your concerns.

SBAR:	RSVP:
- Situation	- Reason
- Background	- Story
- Assessment	- Vital signs
- Recommendation	- Plan

these processes should be followed and staff must be familiar with the hospital processes, particularly in the event of emergency situations such as severe respiratory deterioration necessitating intubation or maternal cardiorespiratory arrest. In this chapter, the considerations for managing a critically ill obstetric patient with suspected or confirmed COVID-19 have been discussed.

References

[1] Scholefield H, Fitzpatrick C, Jokinen M, McGlennan A, Lusa N, McAuliffe F, et al. Providing equity of critical and maternity care for the critically ill pregnant or recently pregnant woman. London: Royal College of Anaesthetists; 2011.

[2] Quinn A, Waldmann C, Materson G, Gauntlett R, Banerjee A, Litchfield K. Care of the critically ill woman in childbirth; enhanced maternal care. London: Royal College of Anaesthetists; 2018.

[3] Vasco M, Pandya S, Van Dyk D, Bishop DG, Wise R, Dyer RA. Maternal critical care in resource-limited settings. Narrative review. Int J Obstet Anesth 2019;37:86–95. https://doi.org/10.1016/j.ijoa.2018.09.010. Epub 2018 Sep 29. PMID: 30482717.

[4] Engström Å, Lindberg I. Critical care nurses' experiences of nursing mothers in an ICU after complicated childbirth. Nurs Crit Care 2013;18:251–7. https://doi.org/10.1111/nicc.12027.

[5] Kinsley J, DeBruyn E, Weaver M. Management of extracorporeal membrane oxygenation for obstetric patients: concerns for critical care nurses. Crit Care Nurse 2019;39(2):E8–15.

[6] Pollock W, Morse K. Chapter 5: midwifery and nursing issues in the intensive care setting. In: van de Velde M, Scholefield H, Plante LA, editors. Maternal critical care: a multidisciplinary approach. Cambridge University Press; 2013.

[7] Knight M, Bunch K, Vousden N, et al. Characteristics and outcomes of pregnant women admitted to hospital with confirmed SARS-CoV-2 infection in UK: national population based cohort study. BMJ 2020;369:m2107.

[8] Zeng H, Xu C, Fan J, et al. Antibodies in infants born to mothers with COVID-19 pneumonia. J Am Med Assoc 2020;323(18):1848–9. https://doi.org/10.1001/jama.2020.4861.

[9] Favre G, Pomar L, Qi X, Nielsen-Saines K, Musso D, Baud D. Guidelines for pregnant women with suspected SARS- CoV-2 infection. Lancet Infect Dis 2020;20:652-653.

[10] British Medical Journal. Coronavirus disease 2019 (Covid-19). 2021. https://bestpractice.bmj. com/topics/en-gb/3000201.

[11] Knight M, Bunch K, Vousden N, et al. UK Obstetric Surveillance System SARS-CoV-2 Infection in Pregnancy Collaborative Group. Characteristics and outcomes of pregnant women admitted to hospital with confirmed SARS-CoV-2 infection in UK: national population based cohort study. BMJ 2020;369:m2107. https://doi.org/10.1136/bmj.m2107. pmid:32513659.

[12] Khalil A, Kalafat E, Benlioglu C, O'Brien P, Morris E, Draycott T, et al. SARS-CoV-2 infection in pregnancy: a systematic review and meta-analysis of clinical features and pregnancy outcomes. E Clin Care 2020;25:100446. https://doi.org/10.1016/j.eclinm.2020.100446.

[13] Talbot L, Maclennon K. Physiology of pregnancy. Anaesth Intensive Care Med 2016;17(7):341–5.

[14] Boyle M, Bothamley J. Critical care assessment by midwives. Taylor and Francis; 2018.

[15] Hirshberg A, Kern-Goldberger AR, Levine LD, Pierce-Williams R, Short WR, Parry S, Berghella V, Triebwasser JE, Srinivas SK. Care of critically ill pregnant patients with coronavirus disease 2019: a case series. Am J Obstet Gynecol 2020;223(2):286–90. https://doi.org/10.1016/j.ajog.2020.04.029. Epub 2020 May 1. PMID: 32371056; PMCID: PMC7252050.

[16] Lapinsky SE. Acute respiratory failure in pregnancy. Obstet Med 2015;8(3):126–32.

[17] Mazlan MZ, Ali S, Zainal Abidin H, Mokhtar AM, Ab Mukmin L, Ayub ZN, Nadarajan C. Non-invasive ventilation in a pregnancy with severe pneumonia. Respir Med Case Rep 2017;8(21):161–3.

[18] Cook TM, El–Boghdadly K, McGuire B, McNarry AF, Patel A, Higgs A. Consensus guidelines for managing the airway in patients with COVID–19. Anaesthesia 2020;75:785–99. https://doi.org/10.1111/anae.15054.

[19] Bordoni L, Parsons K, Rucklidge MWM. Obstetric airway management. Anaesthesia Tutorial of the Week; 2018. Tutorial 393 www.wfsahq.org.

[20] Schnettler WT, Al Ahwel Y, Suhag A. Severe acute respiratory distress syndrome in coronavirus disease 2019-infected pregnancy: obstetric and intensive care considerations. Am J Obstet Gynecol 2020;2(3):100120.

[21] Royal College of Obstetricians and Gynaecologists. Coronavirus infection in pregnancy. Information for healthcare professionals. 2020. Version 12 www.rcog.org.uk.

[22] Shaw P, Duncan A, Voyouka A, Ozsvath K. Radiation exposure and pregnancy. J Vasc Surg 2011;53(1):28S–34S.

[23] LoMauro A, Aliverti A. Respiratory physiology of pregnancy. Breathe 2015;11:297–301.

[24] Soma-Pillay P, Nelson-Piercy C, Tolppanen H, Mebazaa A. Physiological changes in pregnancy. Cardiovasc J Afr 2016;27(2):89–94.

[25] Liu D, et al. Pregnancy and perinatal outcomes of women with coronavirus disease pneumonia. A preliminary analysis. Am J Roentgenol 2020;1:6.

[26] Breslin N, Baptiste C, Miller R, Fuchs K, Goffman D, Gyamfi-Bannerman C, D'Alton M. Coronavirus disease 2019 in pregnancy: early lessons. Am J Obstet Gynaecol 2020;2(2 Suppl):100111.

[27] World Health Organisation. Clinical management of severe acute respiratory infection when novel coronavirus (2019-nCoV) infection is suspected. Interim Guid 2020. www.who.int.

[28] Tolcher MC, McKinney JR, Eppes CS, Muigai D, Shamshirsaz A, Guntupalli KK, Nates JL. Prone positioning for pregnant women with hypoxemia due to coronavirus disease 2019 (COVID-19). Obstet Gynecol 2020;136(2):259–61.

[29] Anselmi A, Ruggieri VG, Letheulle J, Robert AL, Tomasi J, Le Tulzo Y, Verhoye JP, Flécher E. Extracorporeal membrane oxygenation in pregnancy. J Card Surg 2015;30(10):781–6.

[30] Sanghavi M, Rutherford JD. Cardiovascular physiology of pregnancy. Circulation 2014;130:1003–8.

[31] Royal College of Obstetricians and Gynaecologists. Maternal collapse in pregnancy and the puerperium (Green-top guideline No. 56). 2019. https://www.rcog.org.uk/en/guidelines-research-services/guidelines/gtg56/.

[32] Jeejeebhoy FM, Zelop CM, Lipman S, Carvalho B, Joglar J, Mhyre JM, Katz VL, Lapinsky SE, Einav S, Warnes CA, Page RL, Griffin RE, Jain A, Dainty KN, Arafeh J, Windrim R, Koren G, Callaway CW, American Heart Association Emergency Cardiovascular Care Committee, Council on Cardiopulmonary, Critical Care, Perioperative and Resuscitation, Council on Cardiovascular Diseases in the Young, and Council on Clinical Cardiology. Cardiac arrest in pregnancy: a scientific statement from the American Heart Association. Circulation 2015;132(18):1747–73.

[33] Wang D, Hu B, Hu C, et al. Clinical characteristics of 138 hospitalized patients with 2019 novel coronavirus-infected pneumonia in Wuhan, China. JAMA 2020;323:1061–9.

[34] Edlow JA, Caplan LR, O'Brien K, Tibbles CD. Diagnosis of acute neurological emergencies in pregnant and post-partum women. Lancet Neurol 2013;12(2):175–85.

[35] Pelayo J, Pugliese G, Salacup G, Quintero E, Khalifeh A, Jaspan D, Sharma B. Severe COVID-19 in third trimester pregnancy: multidisciplinary approach. Case Rep Crit Care 2020;2020:8889487.

[36] Cheung KL, Lafayette RA. Renal physiology of pregnancy. Adv Chron Kidney Dis 2020;20(3):209–14.

[37] National Institute for Health and Care Excellence. New Covid-19 guideline on acute kidney injury. 2020. https://www.nice.org.uk/news/article/new-covid-19-guideline-on-acute-kidney-injury.

[38] Doyle JF, Forni LG. Acute kidney injury: short-term and long-term effects. Crit Care 2016;20:188. https://doi.org/10.1186/s13054-016-1353-y.

[39] Einarson TR, Piwko C, Koren G. Quantifying the global rates of nausea and vomiting of pregnancy: a meta analysis. J Popul Ther Clin Pharmacol 2013;20(2):e171–83.

[40] Royal College of Obstetricians and Gyanecologists. The management of nausea and vomiting of pregnancy and hyperemesis gravidarum (green-top guideline No 69). 2016. https://www.rcog.org.uk/globalassets/documents/guidelines/green-top-guidelines/gtg69-hyperemesis.pdf.

[41] Heyland DK, Mourtzakis M. Malnutrition in critical illness: implications, causes and therapeutic approaches. In: Stevens RD, Hart N, Herridge MS, editors. Textbook of post-ICU medicine: the legacy of critical care. Oxford University Press; 2014.

[42] Reintam Blaser A, Starkopf J, Alhazzani W, Berger MM, Casaer MP, Deane AM. ESICM Working Group on Gastrointestinal Function. Early enteral nutrition in critically ill patients: ESICM clinical practice guidelines. Intens Care Med 2017;43(3):380–98.

[43] Lewis K, Alqahtani Z, Mcintyre L, et al. The efficacy and safety of prokinetic agents in critically ill patients receiving enteral nutrition: a systematic review and meta-analysis of randomized trials. Crit Care 2016;20:259.

[44] Morelli S, Mandal M, Goldsmith LT, Kashani BN, Ponzio NM. The maternal immune system during pregnancy and its influence on fetal development. Res Rep Biol 2015;6:171–89. https://doi.org/10.2147/RRB.S80652.

[45] sepsis.org. Coronavirus (Covid-19). 2020. https://www.sepsis.org/sepsisand/coronavirus-covid-19/.

[46] Bridwell M, Handzel E, Hynes M, et al. Hypertensive disorders in pregnancy and maternal and neonatal outcomes in Haiti: the importance of surveillance and data collection. BMC Pregnan Childbirth 2019;19:208.

[47] Nolan J, Soar J, Hampshire S, Mitchell S, Pitcher D, Gabboot D, et al. In: Advanced life support manual. 7th ed. London: Resuscitation Council (UK); 2016.

[48] Gates S, Anderson ER. Wound drainage for caesarean section. Cochrane Database Syst Rev 2013;12:CD004549. https://doi.org/10.1002/14651858.CD004549.pub3.

[49] Hinton L, Locock L, Knight M. Maternal critical care: what can we learn from patient experience? A qualitative study. BMJ Open 2015;5:e006676. https://doi.org/10.1136/bmjopen-2014-006676.

[50] Jones ER, Holmes V, Heazell AEP. The use of cold cots following perinatal death. Eur J Obstet Gynecol Reprod Biol 2017;217:179–80.

[51] Lyndon A. Failure to rescue, communication, and safety culture. Clin Obstet Gynecol 2019;62(3):507–17. https://doi.org/10.1097/GRF.0000000000000461.

Chapter 15

Providing end-of-life care during the COVID-19 pandemic

June Frankland, Chris Carter, Joy Notter

Chapter Outline

This chapter describes the end-of-life considerations during the COVID-19 pandemic. COVID-19 has led to an estimated 80,000 deaths in the United Kingdom alone. Although each country uses different criteria to record COVID-19 deaths, across the world this has equated to over 1.9 million people [1,2]. These are in addition to the deaths that occur each year in acute and community settings. The nature of critical care services is such that death and the need for nurses to be able to provide end-of-life care are accepted and essential elements of critical care nursing [3]. However, it has to be noted that as death in a high-technological environment is often sudden and unexpected, unlike palliative care settings, there may have been no time for patients and families to accept and prepare for death. Therefore it is important that in this pandemic where there is such a high incidence of mortality, critical care staff have access to practitioners from palliative care teams to exchange best practice and to seek feedback as appropriate from families regarding the service given.

End-of-life care in the era of COVID-19

Due to the need for personal protective equipment and the restriction of visitors associated with COVID-19, critical care nurses need to adapt accepted end-of-life practices, including communication with patients and families. End-of-life

COVID-19: A Critical Care Textbook. https://doi.org/10.1016/B978-0-7020-8383-9.00015-4

care goals are to keep the patient pain free, comfortable and address any side effects that they may experience, such as nausea, shortness of breath, agitation and emotional distress [4]. During this pandemic, this has proved challenging due to high patient admissions, high bed occupancy and inevitably overstretched resources [5]. However, end-of-life care is an essential part of critical care and must be treated equally and just as importantly as life-saving care. High-quality end-of-life care must include compassion, effective communication, shared decision-making, avoidance of prolonged dying, keeping the patient comfortable and providing respect and dignity whilst taking into consideration the patient's views and wishes [6].

The lay perception of critical care tends to be that interventions save lives; however, it has to be noted that given the severity of illness of patients admitted, an estimated one in seven patients dies [7]. While it is accepted that end-of-life care is a specialist subject in its own right [8], the reality of the figures cited by Pattison [7] are such that it is paramount that critical care staff are thoroughly trained and supported in these situations [9], particularly as during the COVID-19 pandemic, the increased death rates meant that end-of-life care became much more prominent [10].

End of life encompasses all aspects of care for patients who are entering the end stages of their lives, as well as those facing imminent death. Traditionally, this has included patients that may live for weeks, months or up to a year. However, due to the rapid deterioration caused by COVID-19 in many instances, there is little time to prepare patients and their families for death [11]. While every effort is made to maintain symptom control, including shortness of breath, agitation, pain, nausea and vomiting, these treatments require careful monitoring and titration [4]. In a time of pandemic, every effort must be made to meet the rapidly changing individual needs of patients, who increasingly may be conscious throughout the process. A multidisciplinary approach is needed to provide holistic, culturally appropriate patient-centred end-of-life care, but again this may be difficult due to restrictive practices and limited staff, with increasing patient workloads.

Communication

Communication between critical care staff and relatives is challenging [12]. The essentials of communication include establishing a bond of trust, openness and the ability to read non-verbal reactions. Non-verbal cues can indicate the effectiveness of the communication strategies being used [7]. Communication during the pandemic is continually evolving. During the first wave, it became clear that some phone calls were delayed or missed, leading to worry, anxiety, anger and distress on the part of the families [13]. Such problems can be reduced by designated time slots for staff to contact the families, using an identified professional [14]. To further improve communication where appropriate, inclusion of families in management decisions provides an element of shared decision-making, which allows families' perceptions of the aspirations and fears of patients who can no longer speak for themselves to be heard [15].

A wealth of information is offered to relatives, and it is recognized that improvements have been made in critical care to the quality of communication in end-of-life care [16]. During the COVID-19 pandemic, several professional guidelines have been developed on how to communicate with relatives via the telephone. Topics that may need to be addressed include withdrawing and withholding life-sustaining treatments, legal positions, advanced care plans, lasting power of attorney and the patient's own wishes and preferences [17]. Decisions must be high quality, transparent, evidence based and in the patient's best interests, taking into account their values and wishes [3].

With the move to the use of virtual communication, challenges with using technology include the limited prior experience of relatives, particularly if they are elderly, making conversations difficult to start and subtle nuances in facial cues and body language may be missed. Also, families may have had limited or no contact with the critical care team and may not appreciate the severity of the situation. Not all people have smartphone technology; therefore the telephone may be the only way of communicating. It also raises further issues and limitations if the relative has hearing or sight problems, physical disabilities such as poor dexterity and of course possible language barriers [18]. Measures to address these issues include careful planning and consideration of phone or video calls, with an appropriate adult present with the relative at the designated time.

To communicate with critically ill patients can be challenging, particularly if the patient is sedated, intubated and ventilated or has a tracheostomy [19,20]. Speech and language therapists have designed and implemented various forms of communication based upon individual patient's abilities, functions and needs. These include communication boards using pictures and words, speaking valves and electrolarynx boxes for patients with tracheostomies. These are banded under the broad term of augmentative and alternative communication devices (AACDs). AACDs can include all other forms of communication that are used without the use of oral speech [21]. These also include mouthing words, pen and paper, as well as high-tech devices such as tablets with communication apps [21]. Whilst these are usually effective in communication, some limitations were noted, and these include patient fatigue, ability to maintain concentration and restricted movements [22]. However, the use of AACDs has proven to improve patient and family satisfaction, reducing anxiety, stress, panic and frustration [22]. However, communication between patients and staff can prove to be difficult, and every effort needs to be made to avoid miscommunication as this may lead to frustration, isolation and depression [19].

Withdrawal of treatment

The information given in this chapter does not debate the withholding of non-beneficial treatment or the rationing of care when resources are limited, but considers how to provide end-of-life care during the COVID-19 pandemic. It is important to note that different countries have different laws, policies and procedures regarding withdrawal of treatment, but all follow ethical principles, taking note of culture and religion. Therefore nurses need to have knowledge of the healthcare system and laws in which they practice and the policies and procedures used during end-of-life care and, where appropriate, withdrawal of treatment.

As the previous chapters in this book illustrate, critical care interventions can be lifesaving, but in some cases outcome can be uncertain, particularly in this pandemic caused by a new virus. It is accepted that critical care teams communicating rapidly changing situations to patients and families have a very difficult task. For those with a poor prognosis, patients and their families may not have had time to prepare or consider end-of-life decisions. The range of complications caused by COVID-19, and which may lead to end of life, include individuals with severe respiratory failure, comorbidities and critical illnesses [23]. These may lead to withdrawal of life-sustaining treatment, such as stopping mechanical ventilation or administration of vasoactive drugs [24].

Continuing intensive and invasive treatments can prolong suffering and hinder a 'good' death [25]. The need to limit life-sustaining treatments is not unusual [26]; however, the numbers of patients requiring critical care and who deteriorate beyond recovery is unprecedented [27]. The decision to palliate a patient and/or withdraw treatment is first made by the critical care and multidisciplinary teams based on the individual clinical presentation, comorbidities and prognosis of each patient. For each patient and family, ethical considerations must be part of the decision-making process and where possible patients and families must be included in the discussion and where appropriate made aware of the rationale informing the medical decision.

The patient's own views and wishes regarding continuing or extending invasive treatments must be taken into account and adhered to where possible. The rationale for not continuing treatment needs to be clearly explained to the patient (if conscious/appropriate) and relatives. While this is a difficult conversation to have in prepandemic circumstances and is more challenging during a pandemic, it is a crucial aspect of individualized care that must be communicated and documented. Once this has occurred, it becomes the critical care team's responsibility to withdraw the treatments (such as removal of endotracheal tubes, cessation of inotropic infusions) and to initiate and monitor effective symptom control measures, which include medications to relieve distress, pain or agitation [28]. In recognition of the importance of end-of-life care during the COVID-19 pandemic, in the United Kingdom, expert guidelines for critical care teams have been developed [29]; this includes algorithms and criteria for end-of-life care. Application of these guidelines facilitates standardization of care across units.

Withdrawing versus withholding

This is a very controversial and debatable issue, which varies globally, but inevitably includes difficult questions based on ethics, legality, culture, religion and moral practice [30]. Historically, critical care services experienced peaks and troughs of need, for example, during influenza epidemics, critical care admissions increase. However, the COVID-19 pandemic has led to a rapid and unprecedented increase in critical care admissions and workloads have been exponentially expanded, but with limited additional human resources to support the rapidly changing and demanding nursing needs [31,32]. In a pandemic, providing appropriate care for critically ill patients is difficult and stretched to its limits, with the risk that health services can become overwhelmed. In this situation the problems are compounded by limited access to specialized critical care equipment such as ventilators, a lack of available qualified critical care nurses and no availability of routine medications [33].

In this recent COVID-19 pandemic, the limited numbers of viable ventilators were an international concern, which prompted a 'scramble' for ventilators and the equipment necessary for ventilation. This reignited the debate between withdrawal versus withholding treatment [30]. However, this must not be confused with rationing of treatment. As outlined earlier, withdrawal of treatment is based on clinical presentation, which is deemed no longer efficacious. In contrast, withholding treatment is a decision not to commence treatment, also based upon clinical presentation, but including consideration of risk over benefit [30]. This places the intensivist in an ethically, morally and legally difficult position [30]. For families, withdrawing treatment may be perceived differently to withholding treatment. The terminology of both has negative connotations; the withdrawal of treatment may be better understood once the clinical situation has been explained. However, withholding treatment may be perceived as not being willing to offer care or 'to try' [30]. In reality, both decisions are ethical dilemmas for clinical staff, who have to make the best decision they can with the best information they have at the time the decision is made [33].

Grief and loss

Grief is complex, varies with every individual and can lead to depression, anxiety, emotional and psychological distress and post-traumatic stress disorder (PTSD) [34]. Early referral to the multidisciplinary team and in particular palliative care specialists is essential to support both the patient and their family, as it has long been recognized that, for families, a relative dying in critical care is traumatic, but has been even more so during COVID-19 [35]. Factors include restrictions in visiting due to infection control requirements. However, for patients, relatives and staff this has proved to be emotionally distressing, increasing shock and traumatization [35]. Wallace et al. [36] pointed out that this is detrimental to the relatives and has a profound negative effect on their ability to grieve, a process which prior to the pandemic usually began on admission to critical care when staff were able to prepare relatives [37]. For example, prior to the COVID-19 pandemic, with higher nurse-to-patient ratios, relatives were able to spend time with their loved ones, with nursing staff available to talk, comfort and support them as the patient progressed to the end of their life. This builds a rapport between the families and the critical care staff and can help reduce distress as the families come to terms with their loss [38]. In addition, families often comforted and supported each other when in the waiting room [15].

During the pandemic, relatives must utilize their own support network to help them come to terms with the situation. For relatives, being unable to visit and/or remain at the bedside prevents them from witnessing the compassionate and empathic nursing care. To address their stress and anxiety, during COVID-19 critical care staff need to use virtual communication, such as video calls with the relatives while at the bedside of the patient. This allows families to see their relative's clinical condition, to meet the staff providing the care and to gain an insight into the critical care environment. While this is not ideal, it is the best alternative that could be offered during these unprecedented times. Whether withdrawing or withholding life-sustaining treatments, the focus must be on the patient, recognizing that relatives in absentia may struggle to visualize the realities of end of life. This can impact on their grieving process and ability to achieve closure and move forward.

Heart fingerprint project

With families and relatives being unable to visit from the time of admission, adjustment to loss can be even harder. Although staff make every effort to communicate the best they can, this does not compensate for being unable to touch or hold a loved one. Even when a death is expected, bereaved family members frequently experience depression, anxiety, PTSD and the inability to say farewell and the absence of the normal social and cultural support mechanisms for grieving make it more difficult [35]. To provide a physical reminder and keepsake for the relative and their loved ones, the heart fingerprint initiative was introduced by the lead author. The initiative involves creating a heart shape using an ink copy of the patient's fingerprint on a preprinted card, which is then sent to their relative (Pictures 15.1–15.3).

Similar projects exist in other acute settings, for example, organ donation service and neonatal intensive care units, where handprints provide a memento [39]. This hopefully will provide a valued memory during the grieving process for the families of a lost loved one. It is hoped that this will also aid in acceptance and will support the grieving process. Each heart fingerprint is individualized to each patient, making this a unique keepsake. The heart fingerprint provides a lasting physical reminder of the person and is a tangible reminder that can be seen, touched and handed down to future generations, thus keeping the person's memory alive years down the line.

Although a relatively new project, feedback from families has been very positive. Relatives have described it as a lasting memory that they will keep and cherish. Other initiatives include memory boxes, which include locks of hair,

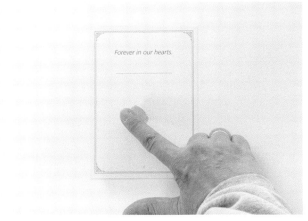

PICTURE 15.1   Place the finger on the card carefully at a 11 to 5 (on clock face) angle.

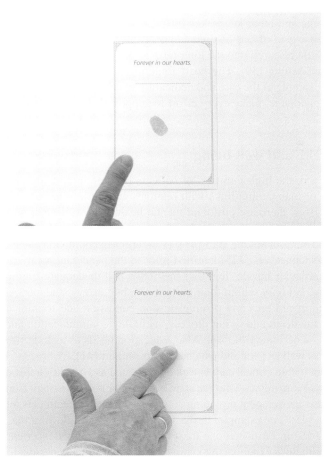

PICTURE 15.2   Place the finger on the card carefully at an 1 to 7 (clock face) angle so fingerprints overlap at the bottom.

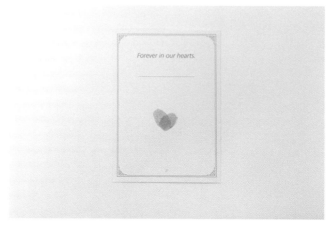

PICTURE 15.3 Heart fingerprint.

knitted items and other keepsakes [40]. Legacy building and memory making can be seen as part of end-of-life and bereavement care. However, to date, there has been little research into the long-term impact of such initiatives in the adult critical care setting [39]. The heart fingerprint initiative described here is an excellent example of the care and dedication of critical care nurses, who even in a time of pandemic, make every effort to support and care for relatives as well as patients.

Staff health and well-being

For staff, too, the high numbers of patients needing end-of-life care, and the challenge of maintaining links with relatives with little time to process events for themselves, there are profound mental health and well-being implications. If not recognized, these can lead to anxiety, depression, PTSD, compassion fatigue and burnout among staff [41]. Difficulties in coping may be exacerbated because, as Goncalves [42] identified prior to the pandemic, many critical care staff, in particular nurses, feel that they have had inadequate training in end-of-life care, not only within their current role but also as students. As a consequence, improved pre- and postregistration education and training for nurses regarding the death and dying process, including communication and counselling skills, is necessary [43,44]. Also, education needs to include strategies for self-care, as well as peer and psychological support [41].

Burnout within critical care is well documented as a condition that does affect many critical care nurses, who are at an even higher risk of burnout from working in an intense environment providing complex and intense treatments for critically ill patients [45]. For example, in the United Kingdom, following the first wave of COVID-19, an estimated one-third of critical care nurses experienced severe burnout, with 86% experiencing symptoms of exhaustion, depersonalization and reduced personal accomplishment [46]. Without additional resources and support provided for staff working within the pandemic, the long-term impact on individual practitioners and their ability to respond to future surges and ongoing delivery of healthcare systems may be compromised [47].

Conclusion

In this chapter, the aim was to give an overview of some of the issues that arise from the need to give end-of-life care during the COVID-19 pandemic. End-of-life consideration is an essential part of critical care provision. While some of the issues discussed arose directly from this pandemic, the principles behind them will translate to other situations where critical care teams are facing a new and ever-evolving clinical situation. Staff health and well-being need to include recognition that with high morbidity, complications and mortality, providing nursing care is both physically and emotionally demanding.

References

[1] Worldometer. Coronavirus cases. 2020. https://www.worldometers.info/coronavirus/.

[2] King's Fund. England has highest excess death rate: the King's Fund responds to ONS international comparisons of mortality data. 2020. https://www.kingsfund.org.uk/press/press-release/excess-death-rate-ons-mortality-data.

[3] Faculty of Intensive Care Medicine. Care at the end of life: a guide to best practice, discussion and decision-making in and around critical care. London: Executive Summary; 2019.

[4] Lovell N, Maddocks M, Etkind S, Taylor K, Carey I, Vora V, Marsh L, Higginson I, Prentice W, Edmonds P, Sleeman K. J Pain Symptom Manag 2020;60(1):e77–81.

[5] Curtis J, Kross E, Stapleton R. The importance of addressing advance care planning and decisions about do-not-resuscitate orders during novel coronavirus. JAMA 2020;12(323):18; 1771–2. https://doi.org/10.1001/jama.2020.4894.

[6] Cordona M, Anstey M, Lewis E, Shanmugam S, Hillman K, Psirides A. Appropriateness of intensive care treatments near the end of life during the COVID-19 pandemic. Breathe 2020;16:2.

[7] Pattison N. End-of-life decisions and care in the midst of a global coronavirus (COVID-19) pandemic. Intensive Crit Care Nurs 2020;58:102862.

[8] Hong S, Cagle J. Comfort with discussions about death, religiosity, and attitudes about end–of–life care. Asian Social work and policy review 2019;13(2):125–208.

[9] Berry M, Brink E, Metaxa V. Time for change? A national audit on bereavement care in intensive care units. J Intensive Care Soc 2017;18(1):11–6.

[10] Swift D. Higher mortality rate in ventilated COVID-19 patients in large sample. 2020. https://www.medscape.com/viewarticle/928605.

[11] General Medical Council. Treatment and care towards the end of life: good practice in decision making. 2020. [London].

[12] Hart J, Turnbull A, Oppenheim I, Courtright K. Family-centered care during the COVID-19 era. J Pain Symptom Manag 2020;60(2):e93–7.

[13] Karlson M, Olnes M, Heyn L. Communication with patients in intensive care units: a scoping review. Nurs Crit Care 2019;24(3):115–31.

[14] Akgun K, Shamas T, Feder S. Communication strategies to mitigate fear and suffering among COVID- 19 patients isolated in the ICU and their families. Heart Lung 2020;49:344–5.

[15] Newcombe V, Baker T, Burnstein R, Tasker R, Menon D. Clinical communication with families in the age of COVID-19: a challenge for critical care teams. 2020. https://blogs.bmj.com/bmj/2020/08/11/clinical-communication-with-families-in-the-age-of-covid-19-a-challenge-for-critical-care-teams/.

[16] Jo M, Song M, Knafl G, Beeber L, Yoo Y, Van Riper M. Family-clinician communication in the ICU and its relationship to psychological distress of family members: a cross sectional study. Int J Nurs Stud 2020;95:34–9.

[17] Parry R, Pattison N &Mannix K. How to have urgent conversations about withdrawing and withholding life sustaining treatments in critical care- including phone and video calls. London: The Faculty of Intensive Care Medicine; 2020.

[18] Annaswamy T, Verduzco-Guitierrez M, Frieden L. Telemedicine barriers and challenges for persons with disabilities: COVID-19 and beyond. Disab Health J 2020;13(4):100973.

[19] Hoorn S, Elbers P, Tuinman P. In: Communicating with conscious mechanically ventilated critically ill patients. vol. 20. 2016. p. 1483–92. 1. 333.

[20] Buheji M, Alhaddad M, Salman A, AlShuwaikh Z, Jahrami H. Hearing the silent voices of COVID-19 patients on mechanical ventilators: the use of augmentative and alternative communication (AAC) approach. Am J Med Med Sci 2020;10(7):457–61. https://doi.org/10.5923/j.ajmms.20201007.04.

[21] Istanboulian L, Rose L, Yunusova Y, Gorospe F, Dale C. Barriers to and facilitators for use of augmentative and alternative communication and voice restorative devices in the adult intensive care unit: a scoping review protocol. Syst Rev 2019;8:311. https://doi.org/10.1186/s13643-019-1232-0.

[22] Santiago C, Roza D, Porretta K, Smith O. The use of tablet and communication app for patients with endotracheal or tracheostomy tubes in the medical surgical Intensive care unit: a pilot, feasibility study. Can J Crit Care Nurs 2019;30(1):17–23.

[23] Vincent J, Taccone FS. Understanding pathways to death in patients with Covid-19. Lancet 2020;8(5):P430–2.

[24] Hoel S, Skjaker R, Haagensen K, Stave M. Decisions to withhold or withdraw life-sustaining treatment in a Norwegian intensive care unit. Acta Anaesthesiol Scand 2014;58(3):329–36.

[25] Ganz F. Improving family intensive care unit experiences at the end of life: barriers and facilitators. Crit Care Nurse 2019;39(3):52–8. https://doi.org/10.4037/ccn2019721

[26] McPherson K, Carlos G, Emmett T, Slaven J, Torke A. Limitation of Life-Sustaining care in the critically ill: a systematic review of the literature. J Hosp Med 2019;14(5):303–10.

[27] Metaxa V. End of life issues in intensive care units. Semin Respir Crit Care Med 2020. https://doi.org/10.1055/s-0040-1710370.

[28] Arya A, Buchman S, Gagnon B, Downar J. Pandemic palliative care: beyond ventilators and saving lives. Can Med Assoc J (CMAJ) 2020;192(15):E400–4. https://doi.org/10.1503/cmaj.200465. Accessed 20/10/20.

[29] National Institute of Clinical Health and Excellence (NICE). COVID 19: rapid guidance for critical care. 2020. https://www.nice.org.uk/guidance/ng159.

[30] Cameron J, Savulescu J, Wilkinson D. Is withdrawing treatment really more problematic than withholding treatment? J Med Ethics 2020;0:1–5.

[31] Vlachos S, Wong A, Metaxa V, Canestrini S, Lopez Soto C, Periselneris J, Lee K, Patrick T, Stovin C, Abernethy K, Albudoor B, Banerjee R, Juma F, Al-Hashimi S, Bernal W, Maharaj R. Hospital mortality and resource implications of hospitalisation with COVID-19 in London, UK: a prospective cohort study. medRxiv 2020. https://doi.org/10.1101/2020.07.16.20155069.

[32] Maves R, Downar J, Dichter R, Hick J, Devereaux A, Geiling J, Kissoon N, Hupert A, Niven A, King A, Rubinson L, Hanfling D, Hodge J, Marshall M, Fischkoff K, Evans L, Tonelli M, Wax R, Seda G, Parrish J, Truong D, Sprung C, Christian M. Triage of scarce critical care resources in COVID-19 an implementation guide for regional allocation: an expert panel report of the Task Force for Mass Critical Care and the American College of Chest Physicians. Chest 2020;158(1):212–25.

[33] Ursin L. Withholding and withdrawing life sustaining treatments: ethically equivalent? Am J Bioeth 2019;19(3):10–20.

[34] Gesi C, Carmassi C, Cerveri G, Carpita B, Cremone I, Dell'osso L. Complicated grief: what to expect after the coronavirus pandemic. Front Psychiatr 2020;11(489):1–5.

[35] Pattison N, White C, Lone N. Bereavement in critical care: a narrative review and practice exploration of current provision of support services and future challenges. J Intensiv Care Soc 2020. https://doi.org/10.1177/1751143720928898.

[36] Wallace C, Wladkowski S, Gibson A, White P. Grief during the COVID-19 pandemic: considerations for palliative care providers. J Pain Manag 2020;60(1):e70–6.

[37] Bandini J. Beyond the hour of death: family experiences of grief and bereavement following an end-of-life hospitalization in the intensive care unit. Health 2020. https://doi.org/10.1177/1363459320946474.

[38] Wood G, Chaitin E, Arnold R. Communication in the ICU: holding a family meeting. UpToDate; 2018.https://www.uptodate.com/contents/communication-in-the-icu-holding-a-family-meeting/print.

[39] Riegel M, Randall S, Buckley T. Memory making in end-of-life-care in the adult intensive care unit: a scoping review of the research literature. Aust Crit Care 2019;32(5):442–7.

[40] Thanh N, Clarke F, Takaoka A, Sadik M, Vanstone M, Phung P, Hjelmhaug K, Hainje J, Smith O, LeBlanc A, Hoad N, Tam B, Reeve B, Cook D. Keepsakes at the end of life. J Pain Symptom Manag 2020;60(5):941–7.

[41] Alharbi J, Jackson D, Usher K. The potential for COVID−19 to contribute to compassion fatigue in critical care nurses. J Clin Nurs 2020;29(15–16):2762–4.

[42] Goncalves S. Death and dying and postmortem care: essential addition to senior skills day. J Nurs Educ 2020;59(1):60.

[43] Tamaki T, Inumaru A, Yokoi Y, Fujii M, Tomita M, Inoue Y, Kido M, Ohno Y, Tsujikawa M. The effectiveness of end-of-life care simulation in undergraduate nursing education: a randomized controlled trial. Nurse Educ Today 2019;76:1–7.

[44] Griffiths I. What are the challenges for nurses when providing end-of-life care in intensive care units? Br J Nurs 2019;28(16):1047–52.

[45] Akgun K, Collett D, Feder S, Shamas T, Shulman-Green D. Sustaining frontline ICU healthcare workers during the COVID-19 pandemic and beyond. Heart Lung 2020;49:346–7.

[46] Ford S. We have asked relevant organisations around the UK to support the Covid-19: Are You OK? Campaign. Nursing Times. 2020. https://www.nursingtimes.net/covid-19-are-you-ok/british-association-of-critical-care-nurses-17-11-2020/.

[47] William RE, Schlak AE, Rushton C. A blueprint for leadership during COVID-19. Nurs Manag 2020;51(8):28–34. https://doi.org/10.1097/01.NUMA.0000688940.29231.6f.

Appendix 1

Case studies and self-test questions

The following case studies and accompanying questions have been designed to test and confirm your knowledge and understanding of problem solving and decision-making when nursing a critically ill patient with suspected or confirmed COVID-19. These questions can be completed before or after reading the relevant chapter. Answers should be considered within the context of your own practice and you should also check regulatory and hospital codes, policies and procedures, as answers provided here are a general guide, and not specific to any one setting or situation.

Pathophysiology of SARS-CoV-2

1) SARS-CoV-2 is an enveloped virus?
   True or False
2) Briefly explain the SARS-CoV-2 virus.
3) Define the term aerosol-generating procedure (AGP).
4) Identify two common AGPs performed in critical care settings.
5) What does the 'R' number mean?
6) What is the incubation period of COVID-19?
7) Identify two respiratory and systemic effects of severe COVID-19.
8) What is the most effective test to identify COVID-19?

Organization of critical care

9) Identify the levels of critical care.
10) In your critical care unit what type of care bundles do you use?
11) List other healthcare professionals involved in the management of critically ill patients and their role.

Assessment and care of the critically ill patient with suspected or confirmed COVID-19

12) 'A' in the ABCDE patient assessment signifies?
    A) Alert
    B) Autonomy
    C) Airway
    D) Acute respiratory distress syndrome

13) A delay in recognizing patient deterioration can lead to?
    A) Delays in treatment
    B) An avoidable admission to critical care
    C) Preventable death
    D) All of the above
14) List three advantages and disadvantages to using an early warning scoring tool in patients with suspected or confirmed COVID-19.
15) List six common methods of monitoring used in critical care?

Case study 1

Mr William James Smith is a 55-year-old man with a past medical history of hypertension and obstructive sleep apnoea (OSA). He presented to the emergency department with a 2-week history of fever, dry cough and shortness of breath. On examination, he denied any chest pain, was found to have tachypnoea (respiratory rate 32/min and SpO_2: 85%), with a non-productive cough, temperature 38.5°C, pulse 105/min and blood pressure 128/98 mmHg. UK National Early Warning Score (NEWS) was 10. Chest X-ray revealed bilateral infiltrates. RT-PCR swabs were taken for SARS-CoV-2.

The initial plan was to start 60% oxygen via a venturi mask, with an aim of maintaining SpO_2 92%–96%. He was commenced on intravenous co-amoxiclav and clarithromycin for community-acquired pneumonia. He was transferred to the admissions ward and was barrier nursed in a side-room.

16) What are the advantages and disadvantages of using Venturi masks?
17) On admission to the ward, assessment of his oxygen saturations are 85% on 60% oxygen via Venturi mask.
    A) Is this reading high or low?
    B) Is any action required?
       Yes/No
    C) If yes, what would you do? If no, what would you do and why?
18) The nurses continued to regularly monitor Mr Smith, and were concerned by his continual increasing respiratory rate (>30 breaths per minute) and low SpO_2 of 88%. He was reviewed by the on-call doctor who increased his oxygen to 15 L/min via a non-rebreath mask.
    A) List three nursing interventions you would provide?
    B) In your setting, how would you escalate your concerns regarding Mr Smith?
19) A trial of conscious prone position is undertaken. Identify two advantages and disadvantages of using this position.
20) Mr Smith continues to deteriorate and his SpO_2 was 72% on high-flow oxygen. An arterial blood gas is taken and shows the following:

Parameter	Result	Normal range
pH	7.32	7.35–7.45
PaO$_2$	4.7 kPa	>10 kPa
	36 mmHg	80–100 mmHg
PaCO$_2$	4.5 kPa	4.5–6 kPa
	34 mmHg	35–45 mmHg

A) What abnormality does this suggest?

B) How should Mr Smith be managed?

21) He has now been reviewed by the critical care consultant and a trial of CPAP is prescribed and he has been accepted for transfer to critical care. List two indications for using CPAP in COVID-19 and what are the possible contraindications?

Day 2 of admission, Mr Smith continues to deteriorate and the decision is made for elective intubation.

22) What precautions do the intubation team need to consider?

23) Mr Smith is intubated with a size 8.0 endotracheal tube. How would you assess Mr Smith's airway patency?

24) What do nurses need to consider when assessing airway and breathing?

25) What do nurses need to consider when assessing a patient's cardiovascular status?

26) When assessing Mr Smith's fluid balance what do nurses need to consider?

27) What is the normal adult urine output that is acceptable?

28) Identify one cause of prerenal acute kidney injury?

29) When assessing neurological status, what do nurses need to consider?

30) When using the Glasgow Coma Scale, the score for responding to voice is?

A) 2

B) 3

C) 4

D) 5

31) You are assessing Mr Smith using the Glasgow Coma Scale, he remains intubated, how would you record this on the observation chart?

A) 5

B) 4

C) 1

D) T

32) Mr Smith is now ventilated on FiO$_2$ 0.5, has tidal volumes of 420 mL and PEEP 8 cm H$_2$O. Peak airway pressure is 30 cm H$_2$O. What are the common modes of invasive ventilation?

33) What does positive end-expiratory pressure (PEEP) do?

34) What is minute volume?

35) What is FiO$_2$?

36) Why are lung-protective strategies used?

37) What are 'lung-protective strategies'?

38) Mr Smith weighs 95 kg, what tidal volume would you expect him to have?

39) During the ward round, the critical care consultant has set a goal of pO$_2$>8 kPa. Mr Smith has had a right radial arterial line inserted, and an ABG is indicated. The results are as follows:

Parameter	Result	Normal range
pH	7.4	7.35–7.45
pO$_2$	7.4 kPa	>10 kPa
	55.5 mmHg	80–100 mmHg
pCO$_2$	5.3 kPa	4.5–6 kPa
	39.7 mmHg	35–45 mmHg

A) What abnormality does this suggest?
B) What would you do?

40) The PEEP is increased to 10 cmH$_2$O and a repeat ABG is performed after 2 hours and shows:

Parameter	Result	Normal range
pH	7.4	7.35–7.45
pO$_2$	9.5 kPa	>10 kPa
	71.3mmHg	80–100 mmHg
pCO$_2$	5.3 kPa	4.5–6 kPa
	39.7 mmHg	35–45 mmHg

A) What does this arterial blood gas show?
B) After a few hours, you are alerted to Mr Smith's ventilator alarming. He appears to be not synchronizing with the ventilator, causing high airway pressure, he looks uncomfortable and the ventilator keeps alarming. What would you do?

41) There is now evidence of ARDS. Mr Smith's fluid balance is positive (1650 mL) and there is a urine output of 50 mL/h. He currently does not require any vasopressor or inotropic medications to support his blood pressure. What strategies could be used to improve his ventilation?

42) Mr Smith continues to deteriorate and it is decided to turn him into the prone position. What does the prone position do?

43) What are the potential complications that may be associated with the prone position that the nurse needs to be aware of?

44) What are the nursing considerations when a patient is in the prone position?

45) Mr Smith has a nasogastric (NG) tube inserted and enteral feeding is commenced. In your setting, what methods are used to confirm NG tube position?

46) What are the benefits of early enteral feeding in critically ill patients?

47) What is the following cardiac rhythm?

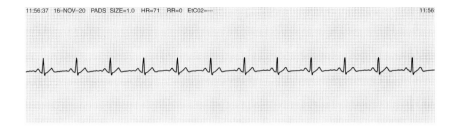

11:56:37 16–NOV–20 PADS SIZE=1.0 HR=71 RR=0 EtC02=----   11:56

48) Mr Smith requires a noradrenaline/norepinephrine infusion due to persistent hypotension and MAP <65 mmHg unresolved by fluid challenges. List five key nursing considerations when caring for a patient requiring a vasopressor infusion.

49) In the event of a cardiorespiratory arrest, what resuscitative treatment can be initiated wearing level 2 PPE?
    A) Defibrillation
    B) Intubation
    C) Chest compressions

50) AED mode has been demonstrated to…
    A) Increase time to first defibrillation
    B) Decrease time to first defibrillation
    C) Decrease preshock pauses

51) The chest compression provider…
    A) Should be swapped every 30 s
    B) Should be swapped at rhythm assessment where possible
    C) Should compress at a rate of 120–140 compressions per minute

52) A reversible cause of cardiac arrest is…
    A) Hypoxia
    B) Hypertension
    C) Tachycardia

53) Ventricular fibrillation is characterized as…
    A) A rhythm compatible with life
    B) A broad complex regular tachycardia
    C) A disorganized rhythm

Case study 2

You are a qualified nurse working in the operating theatres and have been redeployed to critical care during a peak in admissions due to COVID-19. Due to the high number of patients, the critical care unit staffing model involves redeployed staff being allocated a patient, with one critical care nurse supervising a group of redeployed nurses and their patients.

During handover, you are allocated to look after a patient on renal replacement therapy (RRT) by the nurse in charge. You are concerned that you have not had the opportunity to care for a patient on RRT before. You are aware of the staffing levels on the unit and experience of staff on duty, you are seen as the most senior redeployed nurse having had experience of working in critical care over 10 years ago. What would you do?

54) Should you accept handover for this patient?

55) Could you refuse to nurse this patient?

56) How could you manage this situation?

If you are a critical care nurse reading this, consider the questions above from a nurse in charge perspective.

Answers

Case study 1

1) True.

2) The SARS-CoV-2 virus is zoonotic in origin. It requires two key proteins, ACE 2 (a receptor protein that allows the virus to dock to the host) and TMPRRS2 (that activates viral entry into the cell). SARS-CoV-2 binds to the host's transmembrane receptor, ACE2, which is widely found in lung, heart, kidney and gastrointestinal tissue. Once the receptor binds to the cell the cleavage process of the S* protein is activated by the enzyme TMPRRS2, assisting the virion to enter the cell which releases RNA.

3) An AGP is any procedure which can result in the release of airborne particles from the respiratory tract. When treating someone with a suspected or known infectious agent which may be transmitted by droplets, personal protective equipment must be worn.

4) Tracheal intubation, extubation, manual ventilation, for example, ventilation using a self-inflating bag, tracheotomy or tracheostomy procedures (insertion or removal), bronchoscopy, NIV (BiPAP/CPAP), HFNO, HFOV, induction of sputum using nebulized saline and respiratory tract suctioning.

5) The R number used in public health is the estimated average number of infections generated by one infectious person in contact with a population without immunity.

6) 1–14 days

7) Identify two respiratory and systemic effects of severe COVID-19

Respiratory	Systemic
Rhinorrhoea	Fever
Cough (dry or productive)	Fatigue
Sore throat	Ageusia (loss of taste)
Shortness of breath	Headache
Pneumonia	Acute cardiac injury
Ground-glass opacities on chest X-ray or CT scan	Hypoxaemia
	Dyspnoea
Acute respiratory distress syndrome	Lymphopenia
	Diarrhoea

8) Reverse transcriptase polymerase chain reaction (RT-PCR). A limitation to RT-PCR is that although it can confirm the presence of viral RNA it cannot provide information on the presence of infectivity, detection of prior infection or immunity for future infection.

Levels of care

Level 0	Care can be met though acute ward-based care.
Level 1	Patients at risk of deterioration or recently relocated from a higher level of care. Additional input, advice and support from critical care may be required.
Level 2	Patients requiring more detailed observation and intervention including single organ support or post-operative care or patients 'stepping down' from level 3 care.
Level 3	Patients requiring advanced respiratory support and/or basic respiratory support with support of at least two organ systems.

9) Examples include ventilator care bundle, central venous catheter care bundle and tracheostomy care bundle

10) Care bundles commonly used may include: ventilator, tracheostomy, urinary catheter, central venous catheter, neurological, chest drain.

11) Doctors, specialist nurses, dieticians, physiotherapists, pharmacists

12) C

13) D

14)

Advantages of EWS	Disadvantages of EWS
• Supports ward staff to identify patients at risk	• Over-reliance in scores by healthcare professionals
• Ensures full sets of observations are completed	• Lacks clinical judgement
• Score triggers a response, e.g., review	• Limited equipment availability may result in incomplete observations being performed
• Simple and easy to use	• Limited staff may prevent regular vital signs and EWS being performed
• Only basic equipment is required	• EWS are only as accurate as the practitioner performing them
• Requires minimal training	• In COVID-19 EWS may not be sensitive enough to identify patients at risk

15) Respiratory rate, pulse oximetry, heart rate/pulse rate, capillary refill time (CRT), blood pressure (non-invasive/invasive), urine output, neurological status (AVPU or Glasgow Coma Scale) and pupillary reaction, pain score, sedation score, blood glucose levels, daily bloods, fluid balance monitoring, end-tidal carbon dioxide monitoring if intubated and arterial blood gases.

16)

Advantages	Disadvantages
Simple to use	Prevents talking
Widely available	Prevents eating and drinking
	Rebreathing risk at low flow rates
	Can cause dryness of the upper airway

17A) Low

17B) Yes

17C) Nursing considerations include:

- Immediately assess the patient using ABCDE approach.
- Check oxygen is attached and still running at correct rate.
- Check SpO_2 probe position and trace.
- If SpO_2 remains low, increase oxygen.
- Nurse in upright position.
- Consider trialling conscious prone position.
- Call for help and ask for an urgent medical review.
- Increase frequency of assessment of vital signs.

18A) Answers may include:

- Assess patient using ABCDE approach.
- Complete a respiratory assessment: symmetry, percussion, observe for signs of respiratory distress, for example, accessory muscles, see-saw chest/abdominal movement.
- Increase nursing monitoring to 1-hourly vital signs +/– early warning scoring as appropriate.
- Trail of conscious prone position (if not already tried).
- Assess fluid balance status.
- Check intravenous access is patent.
- Consider repeat bloods (e.g., renal profile, full blood count, CRP, ferritin, coagulation screen).
- If cough becomes productive, send sputum specimen for microscopy, culture and sensitivity.
- Request review of intravenous antibiotics.
- Consider updating relatives of situation.
- Consider the effects of oxygen therapy, for example, drying of Mr Smith's nares and mouth, consider regular oral hygiene and check for signs of pressure/skin damage due to the mask and straps on Mr Smith's nose, chin and ears.

18B) Use of a structured communication model such as the Situation, Background, Assessment and Recommendation (SBAR) is recommended. This allows for critical information to be succinctly shared between healthcare professionals. In addition, if using an EWS initiates a response refer to a senior doctor, critical care outreach, medical emergency or rapid response team. If not using an EWS, clinical judgement, objective evidence, for example, vital signs and trends in observations must be used to trigger a call for help. It has to be noted that there is a risk, as this may vary between nurses depending on experience. In consequence, if working with redeployed/junior staff, appropriate supervision and mentorship must be followed.

19)

Advantages	Disadvantages
Simple, can be performed in most settings, e.g. ward	May not be tolerated
Compatible with all forms of basic respiratory support	Depends on stage of disease, e.g., respiratory distress, immediate need for intubation – contraindicated
Requires little or no equipment	Patients with high BMI may not be able to be positioned prone
Potentially improves oxygenation	Difficult to use in 2nd and 3rd trimester pregnancy

20A) Severe hypoxia

20B) Answers may include:

- Check oxygen supply tubing is still attached and still running at correct rate.
- Increase oxygen (if possible), however, remember Mr Smith is already on 15 L via a non-rebreath mask.
- Assess for signs of other potential underlying causes, for example, is there another problem with the respiratory or cardiovascular system? Could an underlying health condition be exacerbated?
- If not done already, increase vital sign monitoring and observation of the patient.
- Assess the need for a bronchodilator nebulizer.
- Consider optimal positioning for effective breathing.
- Urgent medical and critical care review.
- Chest X-ray.
- Prepare for HFNO or CPAP to improve oxygenation.
- Prepare for critical care admission.
- +/– Assemble emergency equipment.
- Reassure and explain all nursing procedures to Mr Smith.
- Consider phoning relatives to provide an update.

21)

Indications	Contraindications
Type 1 respiratory failure	Reduced level of consciousness or unconscious
Atelectasis	Facial injuries
Patient consent	Recent facial/upper gastrointestinal/ upper airway surgery
Can be used as a method of weaning from mechanical ventilation	Pneumothorax

22) Considerations include:
   - Intubation is an AGP, therefore, full PPE including FFP3 and visor as per local and national guidelines is required.
   - Rapid sequence induction (RSI) should be used due to the risk of gastric pulmonary aspiration.
   - Only essential staff should be in the room during the procedure (intubator, an assistant and someone to administer drugs, with a runner outside).
   - Pre-oxygenation should be performed using a two-person technique with a self-inflating bag and appropriately sized mask.
   - The ventilator should be set up prior to intubation and ready to be attached once endotracheal tube position is confirmed.
   - Closed suction catheter should be attached.
   - Depending on local protocol, connections may be taped to prevent disconnection.
   - Grade of intubation and ETT position at lips/teeth should be noted.
   - Continuous end-tidal carbon dioxide should be used to confirm ETT position and monitor ventilation.
   - Auscultation of chest to confirm tube position as long as it does not breach PPE.
   - Confirm ETT position via chest X-ray.

23) Answers may include:
   - Position of ETT at the incisors. This is usually recorded in the notes on intubation and on the critical care observation chart.
   - End-tidal carbon dioxide trace to confirm airway patency.
   - ETT ties are secure and clean.
   - ETT cuff pressure 25–30 mmHg.
   - Depending on PPE used auscultation of the chest.
   - Observation for any signs of pressure damage due to ETT ties, for example, corner of the mouth.
   - Note the Cormack–Lehane or Mallampati classification for grade (difficulty) of intubation.
   - Note the time last suctioned – quantity and description of secretions.
   - Closed suction catheter being used (noting time it was last changed – depending on setting suction catheters may be changed every 24–48 h).

24) Answers may include:
   - Endotracheal tube position and care as outlined in Chapter 6.
   - Observation of the chest for breathing pattern, movement and symmetry.
   - Auscultation as appropriate.
   - Tracheal deviation.
   - Signs of fremitus.
   - Ventilator settings and patient response.
   - Vital signs (respiratory rate, pattern, SpO_2, $EtCO_2$).
   - Arterial blood gas results.

- Chest X-ray to confirm ETT position and any lung pathology.
- Any other tests, for example, CT scan results, microbiology results.
- Sputum type, colour and consistency.

25)

- Heart rate and rhythm.
- Blood pressure (arterial/non-invasive).
- Mean arterial pressure.
- CVP trace.
- Chest X-ray, for example, confirm central line position, signs of pulmonary oedema.
- Arterial blood gas, as this may provide additional information such as electrolytes, haemoglobin level and lactate.
- Blood results including electrolytes, full blood count, coagulation.
- Temperature.
- Patient's past medical history, for example, a patient with hypertension may require a higher BP/MAP to maintain perfusion to the kidneys.
- Any medication that may affect heart rate or blood pressure, for example, beta-blockers, vasopressor infusions.
- Intravenous access (type and location).

26)

- Previous 24-h fluid balance.
- Urine output (aiming for >0.5 mL/kg/h).
- Fluid input.
- Fluid output.
- Overall and ongoing net gain or loss (positive or negative fluid balance).
- In ARDS fluid balance is crucial to optimize lung ventilation.

27) >0.5 mL/kg/h

28) AKI causes include:

- Hypovolaemia, for example, haemorrhage, gastrointestinal losses, excessive diuresis, and third spacing (ascites, pancreatitis).
- Hypotension and low cardiac output states, for example, myocardial dysfunction, arrhythmias.
- Sepsis.
- Effects of positive-pressure ventilation and the use of positive end expiratory pressure (PEEP) may increase intrathoracic pressures, decrease cardiac output, increase in right ventricular afterload. This impairs right ventricular function, which detrimentally increases the systemic nervous pressure, reducing renal perfusion and increasing venous congestion

29) Neurological assessment considerations?

- Glasgow Coma Scale and pupillary reaction.
- Blood glucose level.
- Pain assessment.

- Sedation assessment, for example, Richmond Agitation and Sedation Score.
- Delirium.
- Train of Four if neuromuscular blocking agents are used.

30) B.
31) D.
32) Pressure and volume. Mandatory and assisted.
33) PEEP 'splints' the alveoli, increasing the surface area to improve oxygen uptake and improve compliance.
34) Volume of gas delivery over 1 min. Calculated by:

$$\text{Minute volume} = \text{respiratory rate} \times \text{tidal volume}$$

35) Fraction of inspired oxygen is the amount of oxygen provided. It is normally shown as a decimal number but can be given as a percentage.
36) To prevent/reduce volutrauma and barotrauma.
37) Tidal volume <6 mL/kg, peak airway pressure <35 cmH$_2$O and plateau pressure <30 cmH$_2$O.
38) Tidal volume 6 mL/kg; 6 multiplied by 95 = 570 mL.
39A) Type 1 respiratory failure and hypoxia.
39B) The ABG result is abnormal and should be discussed with the critical care nurse (if not critical care trained) and/or critical care doctors. Mr Smith is not achieving the parameters set (pO$_2$ >8 kPa), therefore, to improve oxygenation, FiO$_2$ and PEEP may be initially increased to increase the amount of oxygen and to recruit alveolar surface area for oxygenation. If this is unsuccessful the I:E ratio may be changed. Finally, the mode of ventilation, prone position used and optimization of sedation and analgesia may need to be reviewed.
40A) Improved oxygenation
  B) Consider the following:
- Assess patient ABCDE.
- Address any factors found, for example, suction needed, bronchospasm.
- Check for signs of mechanical obstruction, for example, endotracheal tube kinking, obstructed due to secretions, cuff leaks.
- Consider deepening sedation (depending on experience and situation).
- Request urgent review by critical care doctors, as the ventilation settings may need to be changed and/or a muscle relaxant needed.
41) Consider the following:
- Assess patient using ABCDE approach.
- Review fluid balance and if not compromising other organs aim for neutral or negative fluid balance.
- A diuretic or fluid restriction may be appropriate, however, the effects should be closely monitored on the cardiovascular and renal systems.

42) Redistributes perfusion. Improves ventilation/perfusion (VQ) matching by maximizing dorsal ventilation.

43) Potential complications include:
- Increased side effects from administration of sedation and/or neuromuscular blocking agents.
- Airway obstruction and displacement of endotracheal tube.
- Vomiting.
- Pressure sores (most cited injury).
- Facial/periorbital oedema.
- IV line displacement.
- CVS instability.
- Ocular injury/corneal abrasions.
- Brachial plexus injury.
- Staff injury.
- Continuous renal replacement therapy line flow problems.

44) Nursing considerations:
- Check head turned sufficiently to avoid kinking ETT and ventilator tubing.
- ECG electrodes need to be positioned on back (reversed).
- Nurse on pressure-relieving mattress.
- Bed head elevation >25°.
- Change head and arm position (swimmer's position) every 2–4 h.
- Consider neuromuscular blockade. Deep sedation (Richmond Agitation and Sedation Score (RASS) –5).
- Check pressure areas, avoid:
- Direct pressure on the eyes.
- Ears not bent over.
- ETT not pressed against the corner of the mouth/lips.
- Nasogastric tube is not pressed against the nostril.
- Male patient's penis is between the legs.
- Urinary catheter secured.
- Any lines and tubing not pressed against skin.

45) Chest X-ray versus pH test. The chest X-ray method is used in some settings, however, most settings confirm position by confirming the gastric pH.
Chest X-ray: bisects carina, below diaphragm near gastric bubble, follows oesophagus.
pH test: Below 4.

46) Prevents malnutrition, supports the immune system, prevents stress ulcer prophylaxis, and maintains healthy bowel function.

47) Sinus rhythm.

48) Nursing considerations:
Only staff who have been trained and formally assessed as competent should care for patients requiring a vasopressor infusion.

Close monitoring:

- Continuous ECG, arterial blood pressure, SpO_2, +/– advanced haemodynamic monitoring.
- Accurate fluid balance (input and output).
- Monitor blood glucose levels.
- Monitor pressure areas, peripheries for blanching/cyanosis, for signs of extravasation.
- Correct prescription/dose:
  - Check sufficient supply of prepared drug.
  - Check accurate drug calculations.
  - Check correct documentation.
- Equipment is functioning properly and plugged in continuous power supply.
- 'Double pumping'.
- Record 12-lead ECG daily.
- Use a dedicated line for administration of vasopressor infusions.
- All syringes containing drugs should be labelled with the appropriate drug label in a place where it can be clearly seen, and include date and time.
- Depending on local policy and protocols, lines will be labelled at the syringe pump and patient end and will include the date and time the line was first used. This will indicate when the line should be changed.

49) A.
50) B.
51) B.
52) A.
53) C.

Case study 2

54) As a registered nurse, you are bound by your professional Code of Practice, therefore, you must work within your competence and scope of practice. You should escalate your concerns to the nurse in charge and/or critical care nurse working with you and discuss your concerns and options.

You need to remember that all nurses are accountable and responsible for their actions. Therefore, you must have the knowledge and skills to perform activities or interventions needed, within the policies and protocols of the organization. By accepting responsibility for this patient you are responsible and accountable for your actions and the patient's safety. As you have identified you have not looked after a patient requiring RRT before, it would be appropriate to request reallocation or to seek an appropriate solution. For example, it may be possible to reduce the number of patients/staff that one critical care nurse is supervising, allowing them to take responsibility for the RRT and support you, to enable you to extend your skills and knowledge. By discussing your concerns with the nurse in charge, they may have a better understanding of your skills and how best to utilize them to meet patient dependency on the critical care unit.

As the nurse in charge you need to consider the points given above, as well as the patient dependency and the skills of the staff available. You should also be able to discuss your rationale for your decision/allocation of patients and listen to the concerns being raised by staff. You should seek to address the concerns as soon as possible to maintain safe systems of working for all the patients' safety and well-being. You should document your decisions and escalate your concerns to your line manager if you are concerned about patient safety and staffing.

55) If you feel you are unable to care for this patient, you must provide a rationale for taking this decision with the nurse in charge. As this situation has occurred during handover, you could discuss this with the nurse in charge immediately and seek an appropriate resolution. If the nurse in charge refuses to listen or seems unwilling to support your rationale, you should escalate your concerns in writing to your line manager. If you refuse care you must follow agreed protocols and policy for your place of work and familiarize yourself with your local safeguarding policies where necessary, in addition to your professional Code, duty of care and protection of the public.

In many countries, professional regulatory bodies and hospitals may have provided specific guidance on being redeployed to unfamiliar areas during the pandemic. Therefore, it is important that nurses know how these additional policies and guidelines relate to their practice. As a nurse you should not be pressurized into taking the patient, if you are not confident or competent to manage the patient.

56) This is a difficult scenario for both the redeployed nurse and the nurse in charge, as providing care in a pandemic means staff are already overstretched. Nevertheless, both must discuss their concerns and provide the rationale for their decisions, as soon as is practicable.

Communication in this situation is critical. As a redeployed nurse it may be appropriate to use negotiation skills and highlight areas of practice you are able to do, for example, recording of vital signs, preparing intravenous infusions, etc. The more time redeployed nurses work in critical care, the more familiar the setting becomes and new skills are developed, therefore, you may be focusing too much on the one aspect you are unsure of (RRT) and in reality you may be able to do more than you initially thought to provide safe care.

As the nurse in charge, if a nurse discusses their limitations with their competence, it may be appropriate to provide practical help, training and supervision as necessary. This may not be immediately possible, in which case the options are to place the nurse with a colleague able to support and guide her through the procedures or to reallocate the patient.

As part of staff development, the critical care unit may have a training pro-gramme for redeployed staff which may help them develop critical care skills. Therefore, it is important for both the redeployed nurse and the nurse in charge to ask if training is possible and/or signpost the nurse to resources available, for example, apps designed with clinical descriptors, e-learning, professional websites and training programmes.

Appendix 2

Glossary of terms and blood tests

ABG See arterial blood gas.

Acid–base balance The balance between the amount of carbonic acid and bicarbonate in the blood, which needs to be maintained at a constant level/ratio in order to keep the hydrogen ion concentration of the plasma at a constant value (pH 7.4)

Acid A substance that releases hydrogen ions when dissolved in water, has a pH below 7.

Acidaemia A condition normally associated with high blood acidity.

Acidosis Condition in which the acidity of body fluids and tissues is abnormally high, therefore, pH <7.35.

Acute kidney injury Kidney failure, rapid onset, usually diagnosed by changes in the serum creatinine concentration or the presence of oliguria.

Acute respiratory distress syndrome (ARDS) Severe respiratory failure caused by widespread inflammation of the lungs.

Aerosol-generating procedure (AGP) Medical procedure resulting in the release of airborne particles from the respiratory tract.

Alkalosis A condition in which the alkalinity of body fluids and tissues is abnormally high, with a pH >7.45.

Apnoea Temporary cessation of breathing.

Arterial blood gas Blood test to determine the gases in arterial blood, normally oxygen, carbon dioxide and nitrogen. Measurements of partial pressures of oxygen and carbon dioxide, together with the blood's pH, gives information on the patient's oxygen saturation within the haemoglobin and the acid–base state.

Arterial line A special narrow-gauge peripheral catheter inserted into an artery for the purpose of continuously monitoring blood pressure and allowing for blood gas sampling.

Atelectasis A common respiratory complication where lung expansion is no longer possible, accompanied by a complete or partial collapse of the entire or lobe of the lung. Different to a pneumothorax.

Bag, valve mask See self-inflating bag.

Base excess Substance that releases hydrogen ions when dissolved in water, has a pH greater than 7.

Beta-blocker Drug that prevents stimulation of the beta-adrenergic receptors at the nerve endings of the sympathetic nervous system, beta-blockers decrease the activity of the heart and may be used to treat hypertension when other treatments have been tried.

Bi-level positive airway pressure (BiPAP) Method of non-invasive ventilation, by using two levels of pressures.

Bougie A hollow or solid cylindrical instrument, usually flexible, that is inserted into the trachea during intubation.

Bradycardia Slowing of the heart rate to less than 60 beats per minute.

Breath sounds Sounds heard through a stethoscope over the lungs during breathing.

Bronchodilator A drug that widens (dilates) the airway passages by relaxing bronchial smooth muscle.

Bronchospasm Narrowing of bronchi by muscular contraction in response to some stimulus, for example, asthma.

Capillary refill time Rapid test performed to assess the adequacy of circulation in an individual with poor cardiac outcome, by pinching the nail bed for 5 s and assessing the time taken for the return of colour once the pressure is released (usually less than 2 s).

Carbon dioxide Colourless gas formed in the tissues during metabolism and carried in the blood to the lungs, where it is exchanged.

Cardiac output Amount of blood ejected by the heart in a minute.

Cardiopulmonary resuscitation (CPR) Emergency procedure for life support, consisting of artificial respirations/ventilations and chest compressions.

Central venous pressure (CVP) An intravenous catheter inserted directly into the subclavian or jugular vein, the tips lie in the inferior or superior vena cava or right atrium. CVP measures right atrial pressure.

Continuous positive airway pressure (CPAP) Continuous pressure of the breathing circuit when a patient is self-ventilating.

COVID-19 A highly infectious respiratory disease caused by novel coronavirus.

Crepitus Cracking sound or grating feeling produced by bone running on bone or roughened cartilage, detected on movement of an arthritic joint.

Cricoid cartilage Cartilage, shaped like a signet ring, which forms part of the anterior and lateral walls and most of the posterior wall of the larynx.

Cricoid pressure Also known as the Sellick manoeuvre. Technique used in which a trained assistant pushes downwards on the cricoid cartilage of a supine patient to aid endotracheal intubation to reduce the risk of pulmonary gastric aspiration.

Cyanosis Bluish discolouration of the skin and mucous membranes resulting from an inadequate amount of oxygen in arterial blood. Can be either peripheral or central.

Dead space Any part of the respiratory tract containing air that does not participate in exchange of oxygen and carbon dioxide.

Diaphragm A dome-shaped muscle that separates the thoracic (chest) and abdominal cavities.

Electrocardiogram (ECG) Tracing of the electrical activity of the heart. Aids diagnosis of heart disease and arrhythmias. Can be continuous (three- or five-lead) ECG monitoring or 12-lead ECG for diagnosis.

Endotracheal tube Tube inserted into the trachea to maintain a patent airway.

Expectoration Coughing and ejecting (spitting out) sputum.

Extracorporeal membrane oxygenation (ECMO) Technique for providing respiratory support, by circulating blood through an extracorporeal circuit to improve gas exchange and perfusion.

Fraction of inspired oxygen (FiO$_2$) Concentration of oxygen in inspired gas. Can range from 0.21 (room air 21%) to 1.0 (100%).

High-flow nasal oxygenation (HFNO) Oxygen delivery system able to deliver up to 100% humidified and heated oxygen at flow rates of up to 60 L per minute.

Hypercapnia The presence in the blood of an abnormally high concentration of carbon dioxide.

Hyperkalaemia The presence in the blood of an abnormally high concentration of potassium, usually caused by the kidneys being unable to excrete it.

Hypoxaemia Reduction of the blood concentration in the arterial blood, recognized clinically by the presence of central and peripheral cyanosis.

Hypoxia Inadequate oxygenation at a cellular level.

Intubation The introduction of an endotracheal tube to maintain an airway in an unconscious or anaesthetized patient. See rapid sequence induction.

Jugular vein pressure The blood pressure in the internal jugular vein, which is an indirect measurement of pressure in the right atrium.

L/min Litres per minute. Unit of measurement used when administering oxygen.

Laryngeal mask airway A supraglottic airway device, inserted into the mouth of a patient requiring artificial ventilation, for example, during anaesthesia.

Laryngoscope A device used to inspect the larynx to aid the insertion of an endotracheal tube.

Magills forceps Long angled forceps for use with a laryngoscope in removing foreign bodies from the mouth and throat of an unconscious patient.

Manometer A device for measuring pressure in a liquid or gas.

mmHg Millimetres of mercury. Unit of measurement used for suction pressure.

Nasopharyngeal airway A curved tube to be inserted down one nostril of an unconscious or semiconscious patient, to sit behind the tongue to create a patent airway.

Non-invasive ventilation Mechanical assistance with self-ventilating patients that do not require intubation.

Non-rebreath mask Device to administer high-flow oxygen to self-ventilating patients.

Oropharyngeal airway A hard curved tube designed to be placed in the mouth of an unconscious patient, behind the tongue to create a patent airway.

P–R interval The interval on an ECG between the onset of atrial activity and ventricular activity.

PaCO$_2$ Partial pressure of carbon dioxide. Amount of carbon dioxide in the blood

PaO$_2$ Partial pressure of oxygen. Amount of oxygen in arterial blood.

Personal protective equipment (PPE) Equipment used to protect an individual's health and safety from exposure to infectious agents including AGPs.

pH A measure of concentration of hydrogen ions in a solution, and therefore of its acidity and alkalinity.

Positive end-expiratory pressure (PEEP) The amount of positive pressure that is maintained at end-expiration and increases the alveolar surface area.

Rapid sequence induction (RSI) Procedure for the insertion of an endotracheal tube, when the patient is at high risk of pulmonary gastric aspiration.

Reproductive 'R' number Used by epidemiologists to estimate the average number of infections generated by one infectious person in a population without immunity.

Respiratory arrest Cessation of breathing, without treatment, quickly leads to cardiac arrest.

Respiratory failure Caused by inadequate gas exchange, described as either Type I or Type II (see below).

Reverse transcriptase polymerase chain reaction (RT-PCR) Test used to detect DNA or RNA and identify if an individual has an active infection.

Rigid suction catheter Special suction catheter used to remove secretions from the mouth. Also termed Yankaeur suction catheter.

SARS-CoV-2 Severe acute respiratory syndrome coronavirus 2. The virus responsible for COVID-19 disease.

Self-inflating bag A device for delivering emergency ventilation by means of a tight-fitting mask or connecting to a laryngeal mask airway or endotracheal tube. It contains a stiff plastic bag, which is squeezed to deliver its gas contents into the patient's airway, when released, it is reinflated from the atmosphere or an attached oxygen supply.

Sputum Material coughed up from the respiratory tract. Its colour, consistency and other characteristics often provide important information affecting diagnosis and the management of respiratory disease.

Stylet A wire inserted into the lumen of an endotracheal tube to give it rigidity during intubation.

Suction The use of pressure to remove unwanted fluids or other material by using a rigid suction catheter (Yankeur) or suction catheter.

Tachycardia Heart rate over 100 beats per minute.

Tachypnoea Rapid respiratory rate >20/min.

Tracheostomy A surgical operation in which an incision is made through the neck into the trachea to relieve obstruction to breathing or facilitate weaning from mechanical ventilation.

Type I respiratory failure Low PaO_2 (<8 kPa) with a normal $PaCO_2$. Caused by pathological processes preventing oxygen exchange in the lungs, without changing the ability to excrete CO_2.

Type II respiratory failure Low PaO_2 (<8 kPa) with a high $PaCO_2$ (>7 kPa). Caused by a problem with the lungs or with the mechanics or control of respiration. Can be described as hypercapnic respiratory failure and often caused by COPD.

Adult blood tests

The following blood test ranges are a guide. Reference ranges may vary slightly between laboratories and countries, therefore, nurses must consult their own national and local standards.

Haematology bloods tests [1,2]

Test	Reference range
Activated partial thromboplastin time (APTT)	26–37 s
Erythrocyte sedimentation rate (ESR)	<10 mm/h
Eosinophils	$0.02–0.5 \times 10^9/L$
Fibrinogen	1.5–4.0 g/L
Folate (serum)	1.5–20.6 µg/L
Haematocrit	
Female	0.33–0.47 L/L
Male	0.35–0.53 L/L
Haemoglobin	
Female	118–148 g/L
Male	133–167 g/L

Test	Reference range
International normalized ratio	2–3 or 3–4
Leucocytes	$4.0 \times 11.0 \times 10^9$/L
Lymphocytes	$1.0–3.0 \times 10^9$/L
Mean cell haemoglobin (MCH)	26–33 pg
Mean cell haemoglobin concentration	330–370 pg/L
Mean cell volume (MCV)	77–98 fL
Monocytes	$0.2–1.0 \times 10^9$/L
Neutrophils	$2.0–7.0 \times 10^9$/L
Partial thromboplastin time	24–34 s
Platelets (thrombocytes)	$143–400 \times 10^9$/L
Prothrombin time	11–14 s
Red cells (erythrocytes)	
Female	$3.9–5.0 \times 10^{12}$/L
Male	$4.3–5.7 \times 10^{12}$/L
White cells total	
Neutrophil granulocytes	$2.0–7.5 \times 10^9$/L
Lymphocytes	$1.5–4.0 \times 10^9$/L
Monocytes	$0.2–0.8 \times 10^9$/L
Eosinophil granulocytes	$0.04–0.4 \times 10^9$/L
Basophil granulocytes	$0.01–0.1 \times 10^9$/L
D-dimers	<500 Units/mL

Biochemistry blood tests [1,2]

Test	Reference range
Alanine aminotransferase (ALT)	5–42 IU/L
Albumin	35–50 g/L
Alkaline phosphatase	20–120 IU/L
Amylase	<300 IU/L
Aspartate aminotransferase (AST)	10–50 IU/L
Bicarbonate (hydrogen carbonate)	24–29 mmol/L
Bilirubin	<21 μmol/L
Calcium	2.2–2.6 mmol/L
Chloride	95–107mmol/L
Cholesterol (Total)	<5.0 mmol/L
Low-density lipoprotein cholesterol	<3.0 mmol/L
High-density lipoprotein cholesterol	>1.2 mmol/L
C-reactive protein	<10 mg/L
Creatine kinase (total)	
Male	30–200 mmol/L
Female	30–150 mmol/L
Creatinine	71–133 μmol/L
Estimated glomerular filtration rate (eGFR)	>90 mL/min/1.73 m^2
Ferritin	
Female	17–300 μg/L
Male	14–150 μg/L
Gamma-glutamyl-transferase (GGT)	5–55 IU/L
Glucose (venous blood, fasting)	3.5–5.5 mmol/L
Lactate venous whole blood	0.7–1.9 mmol/L

Test	Reference range
Lactate dehydrogenase (total)	240–480 IU/L
Magnesium	0.8–1.2 mmol/L
Phosphate	0.8–1.4 mmol/L
Potassium (serum)	3.8–5.0 mmol/L
Protein	60–80 g/L
Sodium	135–145 mmol/L
Transferrin	
Thyroid stimulating hormone	0.2–3.5 mU/L
Triglycerides (fasting)	<1.7 mmol/L
Urea	3.3–6.7 mmol/L

Arterial blood gases [1, 2]

Test	Reference range
pH	7.35–7.45
PaO_2	>10 kPa
	80–100 mmHg
$PaCO_2$	4.5–6 kPa
	35–45 mmHg
Bicarbonate (HCO_3)	22–26 mmol/L
Base excess	–2 to +2 mmol/L

References

1. Blann A. Routine blood results explained. M&K Update Ltd; 2013.
2. Peaete I, Wild K, Nair M, editors. Nursing practice: knowledge and care. John Wiley and Sons; 2014.

Index